Springer Series on ADULTHOOD and AGING

Series Editor: Bernard D. Starr, Ph.D.
Advisory Board: Paul D. Baltes, Ph.D., Jack Botwinick, Ph.D., Carl Eisdorfer, Ph.D., M.D., Donald E. Gelfand, Ph.D., Lissy Jarvik, M.D., Ph.D., Robert Kastenbaum, Ph.D., Neil G. McCluskey, Ph.D., K. Warner Schaie, Ph.D., Nathan W. Shock, Ph.D., and Asher Woldow, M.D.

D0027276

The Brain in Human Aging

Gene D. Cohen, M.D., Ph.D.

VILLA JULIE COLLEGE LIBRARY
STEVENSON, MD 21153

Springer Publishing Company
New York

QP
376
C59
1988

Copyright © 1988 by Springer Publishing Company, Inc.

All rights reserved

No part of this publication may be reproduced, stored in a
retrieval system, or transmitted in any form or by any means,
electronic, mechanical, photocopying, recording, or otherwise,
without the prior permission of Springer Publishing Company, Inc.

Springer Publishing Company, Inc.
536 Broadway
New York, NY 10012

88 89 90 91 92 / 5 4 3 2 1

ISBN 0-8261-5830-7

Printed in the United States of America

58549

To my parents,
upon the excellent advice
of their grandson, Alex.

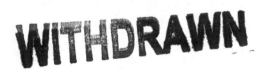

WITHDRAWN

Contents

Preface

The major thrust of this book is to examine a most misunderstood and often maligned phenomenon—the aging brain. Hitherto, the suffering that goes along with mental diseases has been seen as an inevitable part of what it means to be elderly. In older adults disorders ranging from depression to dementia have been mistaken for the norms that we expect to accompany aging. The challenge of perceiving the true nature and potential of the aging brain is now being undertaken by gerontologists, and they are setting the picture straight.

When one takes a good look at the aging brain, myths and stereotypes begin to recede. One sees something rather different from what has been popularly described or expected. Moreover, there is an opportunity to see something *beyond* the real picture of the aging brain alone. By focusing on the aging brain, we can gain a better understanding of human development and disorder across the life cycle—independent of age. Thus, by studying the aging brain we find clues to the nature of mental functioning and to brain disorders applicable to *all* age groups. To overlook the opportunities of research on the aging brain is to pass up possibilities for gaining new insights into relationships between the brain and behavior in general. Research on the aging brain provides us with an additional pathway for uncovering new pieces to the puzzle of the human condition in the face of both illness and health. It is a pathway that science and society largely underappreciated until the fourth quarter of the 20th century (it was, for example, not until 1975 that the National Institute on Aging, the Center on Aging at the National Institute of Mental Health, and the Geriatric Research, Education, and Clinical Centers Program of the Veterans Administration all became operational).

The importance of understanding the aging brain cannot be overstated. Numbers alone make the case when the magnitude and rate of growth of the older population are confronted (U.S. Senate Committee on Aging,

1984; Myers, 1987). At the turn of the twentieth century in America approximately 4% of the population—about 3 million persons—were 65 years of age or older; the average life expectancy was 48 years. By 1975, the 65-and-older age group had grown to 10% of the population—more than 20 million persons; average life expectancy was approaching 74 years. By the mid-1980s there were more than 25 million older adults in America—an elderly population equal to the total population (all age groups) of Canada at that time. America, now, has what is in effect a nation of older persons within its midst. And the same is becoming the situation with all industrialized societies. Moreover, the numbers are still mounting. By 2030 in America, the older population will swell to 21% of the total, or approximately 65 million elderly; this represents an aggregate of persons age 65 and older that is larger than the present population of France.

Both gerontology (the scientific study of aging) and geriatrics (the clinical science addressing health and illness in the elderly) have been advancing in response to the growing number of older adults (Age Page, 1988). As scientists in these fields attempt to look ahead at what avenues of research might be followed during the next 25 years, a lesson that dates back over 25 centuries should be instructive. The lesson comes from ancient Greek mythology and is contained within the myth of Tithonus. Tithonus, a mere mortal, fell in love with Eos, the goddess of dawn. Eos, wanting to live forever with her lover, pleaded to almighty Zeus to bestow the immortality of the gods upon Tithonus. Zeus acquiesced, but while granting immortality, neglected to include eternal youth. As a result, Tithonus proceeds to grow older and older and more and more frail, but without dying. It is extraordinary how this more than 25-century-old myth captures one of the great concerns among gerontological researchers today. This concern is that progress in understanding the mechanisms of aging that leads to increased longevity should *not* outpace progress in improving the quality of the years in later life. Clearly, much of that quality in later life is a factor of the integrity of the aging brain and mind.

More than ever before in history, the capacity of the aging brain and mind to maintain their integrity is now becoming apparent. The significant increase in average longevity combined with improved health care practices in developed nations has resulted in a noticeable rise in the number of older individuals who have aged well—persons maintaining sound minds and bodies well into their later years. These new models of successful aging may well be having an impact on the behavior of our culture that rivals the influence of technology.

For instance, the awareness of powerful technology tends to condense one's time frame, pulling one's focus toward the present where so much is happening so fast. The awareness of positive aging, on the other hand, serves to extend one's orientation to time, pushing one's planning toward the future with its likelihood of a favorable later life. Without models of successful aging, an individual might, in the face of negative expectations, repress images of what it could be like being old. This increases the possibility of "future shock," particularly in a technological society with its pressure on the here and now. But positive expectations of aging permit—indeed encourage—projections of what later life could be like. This adds balance for planning over a much greater period of time, increasing one's personal influence over the shape of one's future. A better understanding of the aging brain should enhance these projections, and this book will discuss the phenomenon of the aging brain from the perspectives of both biology and behavior.

I

The Brain and the Aging Process

1

The Brain Through the Ages

Before examining the brain as it ages, it would be useful to make a quick survey of its evolution over time. First, there is knowledge to be gained from the perspective of the general evolution of the brain, independent of age. Second, information can be derived from studying historical views of the brain, due to aging or otherwise.

EVOLUTION OF THE BRAIN

Our central nervous system, which comprises the brain and the spinal cord, has its evolutionary roots in the *coelenterates,* primitive invertebrates living in the sea some 700 million years ago (the age of the earth is estimated to be about 4.5 billion years, with the first life, thought to be bacteria-like, perhaps appearing around 4 billion years ago) (Garraty & Gay, 1972; Shepherd, 1983). Coelenterates are the earliest forms of animals known to have nerve cells, though they lacked any central control of their rudimentary nervous system. Included among the coelenterates are such species as jellyfish, hydra, and the sea anemone.

Next up the evolutionary ladder in the development of the brain are the flatworms, the first animals in effect to have a head. Flatworms possessed a small brain-like aggregate of specialized sense cells that permitted action by instinct and reflex (The Diagram Group, 1983). But like most animals without a backbone, they were not able to carry out intelligent behavior. This was to come much later with the vertebrates or backboned animals, which first appeared some 400 million years ago. The bony fish which appeared at that time had a central nervous system consisting of a spinal cord which, at its head end, elaborated into a three-part brain. There was a forebrain that dealt with smell, a midbrain that handled vision, and a hindbrain that controlled balance and influenced the viscera or gut. Behavior reflecting true intelligence, however, was still not apparent.

Further evolution saw amphibians (e.g., frogs, salamanders) developing from fishes around 320 million years ago, and this in turn gave rise to reptiles (e.g., dinosaurs, lizards) about 280 million years ago. With the latter, the brain had evolved for life on land. Birds followed next, and then mammals around 200 million years ago.

It is, of course, from mammals that our own species derived, and the arrival of early man was rather recent in evolutionary terms—generally thought to be within the past 5 million years. During this evolution the functions of the three parts of the brain began to shift, and the brain itself became more intricate. Among the later mammals, appearing around 80 million years ago, the forebrain displayed significant development of its outer covering into a new component called the *cerebrum*. Folding of the cerebrum followed, accompanied by the development of the *cerebral cortex* or the outer gray cell area—the locus of higher intellectual brain activity. The most advanced mammals were the primates, including monkeys, apes, and, eventually, man. *Homo sapiens*—man, as we know him today—dates back only about 50,000 years.

PLASTICITY OF THE BRAIN

How does this brief review of the evolutionary development of the brain relate to our understanding of the brain as it ages? To begin with, one needs to think about the ramifications of 700 million years of nervous system development. Clearly, we are looking at an enormous time interval of refinement, adaptation, and ever greater capacity as the brain develops. What is nonadaptive falls out in evolution. The ability to adapt or to compensate for change sets the stage for resiliency and endurance. Historically, until only very recently, scientists have not seen the brain of modern man as being very resilient physically—despite 700 million years of evolution. It should not be surprising then that the aging brain has been seen as even less capable of adapting or compensating for change. Significant new views, however, are now beginning to emerge about the potential of the brain to respond to even serious damage (Cotman & Holets, 1985; Kordower, Dean, White, and Marciano, 1988). And these views of *brain plasticity,* as this phenomenon is referred to, are carrying over to the aging brain as well. Indeed many of the most dramatic examples of the capacity of man's brain to adjust to physical "insult" are found in the elderly. We will return to the discussion of the *plasticity* of the aging brain in considerably greater detail in Chapter 3.

THE MISEMPHASIS ON BRAIN SIZE

While the development of brain resiliency over evolutionary time has been inadequately studied, our concentration on studying brain size has often been misleading. Brain size needs to be put into perspective from an evolutionary standpoint; it also needs to be better understood in the aging of a single individual. Typically, with regard to brain size, many have thought "if it's bigger, it's better." To a significant extent this is true. But there are a number of important exceptions (Asimov, 1965; Restak, 1980; Sagan, 1977).

By no means does man have the largest brain. Whales and elephants, for example, are the largest mammals, and their brains are massive, reaching 9000 g (nearly 20 lb) in whales and 6000 g (about 13 lb) in elephants. A human brain weighs about 1400 g on the average (a little over 3 lb). Of course, one has to take into consideration the amount of total body mass the brain has to regulate to put these brain sizes into a proper frame of reference. Hence, while the largest elephant brain may be 4 times the size of the largest human brain, the elephant's overall size is 100 times that of a human's. This gives an improved brain/body ratio of 25 to 1 comparing humans to elephants; and 250 to 1 comparing humans to the largest whales. The sperm whale, meanwhile, has a brain 100 times the weight of the largest dinosaur brain. But before we dismiss larger brains than humans' as artifacts of larger bodies, consider the dolphin. Some dolphins are no larger than man and yet have bigger brains, with weights up to 1700 g (nearly 3¾ lb). Moreover, the convoluted feature of man's brain can also be seen with dolphins, who possess even greater convolution. This is not to say that dolphins are smarter. On the contrary, they are not.

What might explain why dolphins are less intelligent than humans, despite their larger and more convoluted brains? It has been suggested that the internal organization of these brains differ, just as the internal organization of different computers of similar size can differ widely. Here the computer analogy may be quite helpful for reexamining the "bigger is better" scenario. We continue to witness reductions in the sizes of various computers while they gain greater capacity and flexibility. The difference often lies in increased and more sophisticated interconnections among the pathways and integrating systems of the computer. So, too, with the human brain, where we are now starting to get a better picture of the enormous number of neurons (literally thousands) among which a single nerve cell in the brain can communicate (the human brain is estimated to have as many as 16.5 billion nerve cells or neurons in the cerebral cortex alone) (Adams, 1980). Part of the difference in the internal organization of a dolphin brain may be the likelihood of its being more involved with regulating "lower functions," such as dealing with sound and motor skills essential to negotiating the sea, as opposed to "higher functions," such as abstract thought and memory.

Among humans themselves there is considerable variation in brain size that is not reflected in differences in intellectual abilities. The brain of an adult would have to be under 1000 g in weight for impaired intellectual functioning to be predicted on the basis of brain size alone. Also, on the average, women's brains weigh 10% less than men's, though no differences in overall intelligence have been detected. The brain weight differences probably can be attributed to differences in total body mass among the sexes, with overall brain/body ratios being similar. Moreover, during the past 350 years the brains of various talented intellectuals have been weighed and subsequently compared. The nineteenth century Russian novelist Ivan Turgenev was reported to have had a brain weighing in excess of 2000 g, while the equally gifted French novelist Anatole France who won a Nobel Prize in literature in 1921, was reported to have a much smaller than average brain, weighing less than 1200 g. Many peoplè have had very large brains who were no Einsteins; Albert Einstein himself did not have a remarkably large brain.

For individuals then to possess great intelligence with brains of average or subaverage size suggests in part that there may be significant tissue reserve in the brain, just as there is in other organs. It also suggests that anatomy and structure are not the only determinants of function; chemistry and physiology also need to be reckoned with in explaining the nature of intellectual and other behaviors (see Chapter 2). For instance, an anatomical change may take the form of a brain ending up with fewer cells, but those cells present might have the capacity to compensate for size and respond either by producing more of a given chemical or else by needing to receive less of that chemical to carry out their essential functions. Brain resiliency might be explained in this manner (see Chapter 3).

BRAIN SIZE AND AGING

Returning to the matter of brain size, this past century has witnessed an extensive number of studies measuring brain weight and taking into consideration age factors. A review of these studies has found that the brain reaches its maximum weight at approximately 20 years of age, and that a linear regression of 90 to 100 g occurs by the ninth decade (Brody, 1978; Brody, 1987). Hence, most normal aging brains appear to undergo less than a 10% decrement in size over the life cycle. This would still put the average normal 80-year-old brain at a greater weight than that of the Nobel Laureate, Anatole France. What about France's intellectual performance as he approached 80 with his less than 1200 g brain? Anatole France lived until he was 80, and he was still writing accomplished works up until his death (*Britannica,* 1985c).

Moreover, one does not have to be a genius to display continued high intellectual performance at an advanced age (see Chapter 2). Studies of healthy aging individuals of average intelligence, for example, have found that they continue to expand their vocabulary well into their 80s if not beyond (Granick & Patterson, 1972). Thus, just as having huge brains does not make animals like elephants and whales intellectual giants, a smaller than average human brain can still effect a big intellectual package. Similarly, normal decrement of brain size with aging need *not* interfere with ongoing intellectual achievement or even growth in various areas (see Chapter 2). The other side of this discussion is that, for too long, conclusions about the significance of brain size from both evolutionary and aging viewpoints have fostered negative expectations toward those with aging brains. The story is much more complicated, and new facts are coming in.

2
The Biology of the Normal Aging Brain

What is normal? Colarusso and Nemiroff (1981) in focusing on the mind and behavior over time struggled with this question, offering the following definition of *normal:* "that mental activity and behavior which, based on current knowledge, falls within the broad range of predictable expectation, fulfills developmental potential, and is adaptive to the society in which it occurs."

But the concept of normality is easily clouded, particularly in the context of aging. Clouding occurs when normality is defined as "usual," as "conforming to the standard"; it also occurs when "not abnormal" is offered as a definition (*The Random House Dictionary of the English Language,* 1971). Findings from gerontologic research dramatize the divergency with which what is usual and what is abnormal have been described in association with aging (Rowe & Kahn, 1987). While significant strides have been taken in distinguishing illness (the abnormal) in later life from normal concomitants of the aging process, less progress has been made in defining what is usual. Further confusing the issue is the tendency to *expect* functional decrement in the aging, in every parameter under consideration. This expectation of decline has the unfortunate effect of distorting almost every aspect of the normal aging brain that we examine. Typically, what is diminished is pointed up, while what is strengthened is selectively ignored. This illustrates the usefulness of the Colarusso and Nemiroff definition—that it considers normality within the changing biopsychosocial context of the aging process.

TOOLS FOR STUDYING THE AGING BRAIN

Contemporary tools for studying the aging brain range from high tech computerized imaging techniques that take pictures of what is going on inside the skull to sophisticated psychological tests that permit us to probe one's thinking processes.

Brain Imaging Techniques: CT (CAT), MRI (NMR), and PET Scans

In the last quarter of the twentieth century the introduction of the CT or CAT (computerized axial tomography), the MRI (magnetic resonance imaging) or NMR (nuclear magnetic resonance), and the PET (positron emission tomography) scanning techniques brought about a revolution in brain study (Andreasen, 1988; Dyer & Spragens, 1985; Rosse & Morihisa, 1988; Solomon, 1985). These instruments achieved this by bringing a new capacity for monitoring the brain, and hence a heightened interest in its study. Interest in the aging brain grew especially.

Earlier x-ray techniques had three major shortcomings: (1) their inability to give much information about soft tissues of the body such as the brain (they are most useful with bones); (2) their inability to provide three-dimensional information that could precisely determine the location of a structure or lesion (i.e., the coordinates of its position) within a specific organ; (3) their inability to convey information about the *activity* or metabolism of the structures they reveal. The new imaging techniques have completely changed all of this. The CAT scan provides pictures of the soft tissues and organs within the body along with depth of field data for better localization of a particular structure; the MRI can do this even more dramatically. While the CAT scan and MRI provide brand new anatomical or structural information about body organs, the PET scan enables one to know how active or inactive a particular organ or part of that organ is at a given point in time (it is not clear how much information about activity the MRI may eventually be able to provide).

A CAT scan, for example, is able to identify and precisely locate a brain tumor, but because it gives no information about the activity of tissue it cannot indicate whether the subject is dead or alive. With the PET scan a viewer does know whether the subject is living or not and also receives a color-coded picture showing the level of activity of the tumor and the surrounding tissues. MRI gives an excellent picture of the cerebral cortex of the aging brain for purposes of comparing it anatomically to that of a younger adult, but the PET scan can compare levels of activity within a young and an aging brain in response to the same stimulus.

Basically, the CAT scan evolved from mating computer technology with the x-ray machine, and brought a Nobel Prize to those who developed the mathematical calculations behind it. CAT scanning involves x-raying the brain from multiple angles. An electronic detector, together with an x-ray device delivering very small amounts of x-rays, are rotated around the patient's head. Different angles of rotations provide different scans. Responses from the detector are then fed into a computer, which analyzes and integrates the x-ray data from the many different scans. Cross-sectional images of the brain are then created. By knowing which cross section—i.e., which slice of the brain is being examined—the researcher or clinician can determine the precise location of the structure being studied. It is this ability to get an image at a specific plane or layer that is the nature of *tomography,* and it is tomography that gives the greater clarity and detail of a CAT scan as compared to a conventional x-ray, which cannot separate out different layers and therefore blurs many structures together.

MRI and NMR refer to the same technique. Because many incorrectly inferred from the reference to "nuclear" in *n*uclear *m*agnetic *r*esonance that NMR involved the use of x-rays, the term MRI or MR is now being increasingly used. MRI does *not* involve x-rays; radio waves are used instead. Radio waves are beamed to specific tissues of a patient's body in conjunction with a strong magnetic field. The nuclei within the atoms of the respective tissues in turn give off electromagnetic signals that are translated by a computer into vivid images of the area under inspection. The brain's different anatomical components (e.g., nerve cell layers, blood vessels, cerebrospinal fluid chambers, etc.) are made up of different atoms whose nuclei respond to the MRI by emitting distinct signals; computerized analysis of these signals produces an image providing excellent differentiation of the respective brain parts. It has been said MRI scanning "is better than working with a cadaver because it reveals more anatomic information than can be gained at the dissecting table" (Bryan, 1985). Efforts are also underway to use the MRI for evaluating chemical activity within tissues under observation, which would make this technique valuable not only for studying structures, but for studying metabolism as well.

Though it was not until 1977 that the first MRI for imaging the body was constructed, the theoretical basis for MRI was established in the 1940s by physicists Edward Purcell and Felix Block in the United States, work that won these two scientists a Nobel Prize in 1952. Contributions from MRI scans to the improved understanding of the aging brain are likely to be better than those of CT scans, due to the greater delineation of detail that is possible, and because of the future likelihood of MRI being able to provide metabolic as well as anatomic data.

The PET scan represents another revolutionary breakthrough because of its capacity to measure brain activity and metabolic phenomena. This technique, however, because of its complexity (e.g., it requires a 20-ton cyclotron), remains essentially a research tool, with relatively few such machines in existence. The PET scan combines two technologies: (1) the use of radioisotopes (radioactively tagged elements whose emissions of positrons can be detected radiographically or electronically, thereby allowing the path and activity of these chemicals to be tracked), and (2) the use of computerized tomographic techniques as in CAT scanning that allows the isotopes to be studied and viewed at different sections of the brain.

Glucose, which is utilized by brain tissue for energy, can be radioactively tagged, injected, and traced using PET technology. The researcher can then assess the activity of different brain tissues responding to a given stimulus as a factor of the glucose used for the energy to make the responses. An area of the brain that is more active at a given moment uses a greater amount of the tagged glucose. Accordingly, greater photon emission will occur at that site, resulting in a greater degree of metabolic activity being detected and translated into a color-coded image.

For example, if one is exposed to visual stimuli with the eyes open, the occipital lobe of the brain, which processes incoming visual stimuli, will appear red on the PET scan, reflecting significant metabolic activity due to high glucose utilization in that part of the cerebral cortex. If the eyes are closed, the occipital region of the brain will appear blue on the PET scan, indicating a very low level of glucose utilization and activity. By studying such responses to brain stimuli, scientists are attempting to discover fundamental new insights into the nature of our thinking and intellectual processes. Application of PET technology to the aging brain has acquired rigor and momentum only since the early 1980s.

Test Results and Aging

While PET, MRI, and CAT scans are among the newest and most revolutionary tests helping investigators unlock the mysteries of the aging brain, there are a number of other important tests also being used in this research. These run the gamut from the biological to the psychological, from blood flow studies to depression scale measures. The electron microscope, which can magnify minute structures in excess of ×100,000, is called upon for multiple purposes, including the counting of aging brain cells. The electroencephalogram (EEG), which measures the brain's electrical activity, provides important information in comparing the normal aging brain with brains affected by different diseases in later life. A range of biochemical techniques is also available to analyze the chemical composition of different parts of the brain and the composition of brains of different ages.

While tools and techniques for studying the structure and metabolism of the aging brain continue to grow more sophisticated, tests for assessing cognitive, psychological, and social functioning in later life are similarly improving. The latter range from clinical examinations to community surveys that investigate intelligence, learning, memory, problem solving, attitudes, mood, behavior, stress, coping, adaptation, personality, life satisfaction, and other aspects of one's internal and external environments.

The tools for studying the aging brain, in short, have been applied to examine both behavior and biology in later life; these tests and techniques have also been used to research relationships *between* biology and behavior with aging. The balance of this chapter will concentrate on the biology of the aging brain. Chapter 3 focuses on the subject of behavior and the aging, and Part I ends with Chapter 4, on the interrelationships between the aging brain and the aging body.

THE BIOLOGY OF THE AGING BRAIN

Brain Cell Changes and Aging

Anatomically, we know that, on the average, the brain of a person in his or her 80s weighs about 10% less than the brain of someone the same size and sex in his or her 20s. But we also know that the brain, like most organs, has reserve capacity, with more than 15 billion neurons alone. People can sustain substantial loss in other complex essential organs (e.g., kidneys, liver, pancreas) and still function quite adequately; a 10% loss in these organs would not likely be apparent clinically (witness the fact that one can live a basically normal life with only one kidney—a 50% loss). In the aging pancreas, its enzyme lipase, which is involved in the body's metabolism of fats, can decrease in output by 90% before clinical consequences become apparent. Such variability of the body's chemistry, within the boundaries of normal functioning, should be kept in mind when looking at neurochemical variations in the aging brain. Our perspective on a 10% difference is further enhanced when we remember that brains of women are typically 10% smaller than brains of men, without differences in overall intellectual capacities. Moreover, the historical studies revealed that the brains of geniuses have differed in size by as much as 40%, while some geniuses have had brain weights well over 10% less than persons of average intellect.

Curiously, the aging process appears not to affect all brain regions equally. Even within a given region of the brain, different types of nerve cells may show marked differences as a factor of age. The cerebral cortex, for example, is much more affected by cell loss with aging than is the brain stem (see Figure 2.1). Some brain cell nuclei (masses of gray matter, composed of nerve cells) do not show cell loss with aging (e.g., the facial nerve nucleus located in the pons and the ventral cochlear nucleus located at the junction of the brain stem and the cerebellum), while others (the locus ceruleus located in the pons and the substantia nigra located in the midbrain) manifest significant loss of cells with advancing age (Brody & Vijayashankar, 1977; Carlsson, 1985a).

Findings from other research have led to the question as to whether neurons of the human cerebral cortex are really lost during aging (Haug, 1985). Here, morphologic changes in gross anatomy, specifically atrophy, are attributed more to nerve cell shrinkage than to loss. The positive ramification of this line of investigation is that cell shrinkage is potentially more modifiable than cell loss, in efforts to restore or improve cerebral functioning in later life.

Linkages between anatomic structures and physiologic functioning in the brain have become better understood with the identification of neurotransmitters, chemical substances that enable communication to occur between nerve cells. The locus ceruleus is a site active with neurons producing the neurotransmitter norepinephrine, and the substantia nigra an area of nerve cells producing the neurotransmitter dopamine. Interestingly, it is

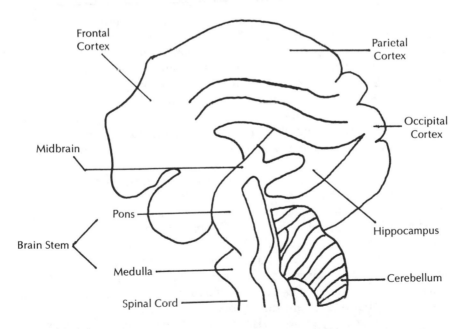

Figure 2.1 Longitudinal section of brain from front (*left*) to back (*right*).

not until the seventh decade that the changes in these two sites become more pronounced, as opposed to a gradual reduction in cells spread out evenly over the decades; the identification of a particular point in time as to when a change becomes more manifest has fostered "clocks of aging" theories, to be discussed in Chapter 10.

Researchers have viewed brain-region and decade-of-life differences in falling cell counts of varying types of neurons as suggesting the existence of one or more age-related factors in the brain that are influencing these changes (Carlsson, 1985a). In other words, certain factors or substances may be activated or produced in the brain that induce brain cell changes associated with aging. These factors and their nature are speculative—as is what might be controlling their action or prompting their appearance— but they are postulated to exert a general, nonspecific influence on nerve cells, affecting cell bodies and nerve terminals alike. Neurotransmitter-like substances with metabolism influencing capacities are candidates. Theoretically, if such factors do exist and are identified, then they could conceivably be manipulated through chemical or drug interventions. Such considerations are explored further in the discussion of resiliency and repair of the aging brain in Chapter 8.

Compensatory Physiologic Events and Aging

Time and again physiologists caution us about not looking at bodily changes in isolation. We are reminded that decrements or increments of a given physiologic activity are typically responded to through a feedback loop by a counterbalancing reaction. This applies equally strongly to the brain. The lesson is too often forgotten with the *aging* brain, as if aging excludes compensatory physiologic events that contribute to the organism's dynamic equilibrium, which plays a major part in maintaining health. What has been found upon further investigation of sites where loss of norepinephrine-producing and dopamine-producing neurons occurs illustrates this point.

With a decline in the number of these neurotransmitter-producing nerve cells, feedback mechanisms operate to stimulate the remaining neurons to increase their synthesis and release of the respective neurotransmitters. Supporting this conclusion have been findings at such sites of constant—if not slightly greater—levels of the metabolites of the affected neurotransmitters (Carlsson, 1985b). That the levels of these *metabolites* (active breakdown products formed by enzymes interacting with the neurotransmitters) are maintained *independent* of aging in the normal aging brain, indicates that reactions are taking place to compensate for declines in specific populations of nerve cells. Another compensatory mechanism appears to be creating increased sensitivity of the receptor sites upon which the neurotransmitters act. Increased receptor site sensitivity results in greater potency for individual neurotransmitter molecules, causing fewer molecules to be needed to trigger the same events.

Increased receptor site sensitivity is thought to partially explain altered psychotropic drug responses in the elderly. Psychotropic medications are believed to achieve their clinical effects through their pharmacokinetic effects on specific receptor sites. If a specific group of receptors requires less chemical stimulus to trigger a response, then less of the given drug that acts on these receptors is required to have an effect. This is one likely reason why the elderly often require less medication than younger adults. The other side of this coin is that if less of a drug is necessary to achieve its desired effect in later life, then using the same amount of the medication in an older person that one gives to a younger one may result in toxic side effects in the elderly individual. This understanding of the normal aging brain is leading to improved management of medications in elderly patients. It is also adding to our knowledge of how external pharmacologic interventions can facilitate compensatory neurochemical processes when internal physiologic mechanisms falter.

Neurochemical Changes and Aging

As our ability to assay brain chemistry has rapidly progressed, we have identified an increasing number of neurochemical substances. Gerontology studies the impact of aging on these substances along with the converse—the impact of these substances on aging. Aging in the central nervous system, as elsewhere in the human body, appears to involve a series of highly regulated, selective changes. Some age-associated changes are interrelated and have been described as "a cascade of interactions which involve hormones, neurotransmitters, and other physiologic factors" (Finch, 1985a). Evidence is mounting that understanding these interactions increases the potential to intervene and alter events that accompany aging—to influence resiliency and plasticity of the brain and behavior with aging (Morley, 1986).

Returning to the neurotransmitters, current hypotheses about memory, thinking, emotion, and behavior have focused on a specific group of these chemicals: norepinephrine, serotonin, dopamine, acetylcholine, and gama-aminobutyric acid (GABA) (Morley, 1986; Rossor, 1985). *Norepinephrine* and *serotonin* are associated with mood regulation. *Dopamine* is primarily linked with motor coordination; a deficiency of this neurotransmitter is found in Parkinson's disease, while an excess has been identified with psychotic symptoms. *Acetylcholine* appears to play a major role in memory and intellectual functioning, and has been found to be deficient in Alzheimer's disease. *GABA* may function as an integrater of different sets of neurons, linking dopamine and acetylcholine pathways, and those of norepinephrine and serotonin; it may also influence symptoms of anxiety, and has been shown to be reduced in Huntington's disease. All of these neurotransmitters are reported to be somewhat diminished with aging, though compensatory mechanisms in healthy older individuals appear to prevent the changes from resulting in clinical symptomatology.

In the disease states just mentioned, pathological processes are at work that lower the levels of these neurotransmitters below various thresholds, at which point disorders, as distinguished from the aging process, emerge. The normal lowering of neurotransmitter levels may contribute to the increased vulnerability to certain psychological and organic mental disorders associated with advanced age, but these normal variations alone do not cause the respective illnesses.

Other neurochemicals are being identified and their relation to aging is under study. Large numbers of neuron-produced *peptides* (protein derivatives) have been discovered in different locations of the brain, these substances appearing to act as neurotransmitters or neuromodulators of various physiologic events. Research is still rudimentary in this area. Nonetheless, one neuropeptide in particular has been the focus of much investigation. *Somatostatin* has elicited interest because fairly constant levels of it have been found in normal aging brains, as opposed to deficits of it being reported in both Alzheimer's disease and the dementia that can accompany certain patients with Parkinson's disease (Morley, 1986; Rossor, 1985).

Here again, to the extent that neurochemical actions and reactions are understood in the aging brain, the potential to maintain homeostasis or physiologic equilibrium with external interventions when internal mechanisms are failing is expected to be enhanced.

Findings from CT and PET Scans of the Aging Brain

Findings from neuroimaging (CT and PET) studies of the aging brain highlight discrepancies between anatomy and physiology—between structure and function in later life. These findings further illustrate the reserve capacity of the aging brain. Because investigations of the aging brain are further along with CT and PET studies than with MRI research, the focus will be on the former two scanning techniques.

CT scans, for example, show changes suggestive of brain tissue shrinkage in normal elderly subjects. But these anatomic changes typically are not accompanied by functional correlates in the form of compromised intellectual capacity or behavioral aberrations (Bryan, 1985). Shortcomings in looking at gross anatomical brain changes as the explanation or primary basis for changes in how an older person functions are further illustrated in the case of Alzheimer's disease. Changes in the gross anatomy of the brains of those with Alzheimer's disease have long been of interest, for both diagnostic and research purposes. Clinically, if one could document characteristic patterns or degrees of brain atrophy in Alzheimer's disease, then brain imaging techniques like CT scans could be potentially of great value in diagnosing the disorder. While such studies are still in progress, CT scans of a number of individuals with Alzheimer's disease—particularly in the early to middle stages of the disorder—cannot be differentiated from CT scans of normal aging brains. Conversely, a CT scan revealing moderate cortical atrophy may not be accompanied by apparent gross functional deficits in an elderly individual (Bryan, 1985; de Leon, Ferris, & George, 1985). CT scans, though, do reveal the presence of other diseases of the aging brain, including tumors, strokes, subdural hematomas resulting from trauma, and the like; hence, CT scans help in differentiating Alzheimer's disease from these other disorders.

PET scan studies, though at an early stage of development, are adding information about the aging brain. A major emphasis of these early studies has been on comparing glucose metabolism (as a reflection of brain activity) between normal older and younger adults, and between healthy elderly individuals and those with Alzheimer's disease. There has been a fair amount of variation in the reports on normal aging brains. Nonetheless, some of these studies have found no specific glucose metabolism changes in normal aging, that is, *the metabolic activity of brains of healthy older adults has very closely resembled that found in younger persons* (de Leon, Ferris, & George, 1985). Other research has reported that cerebral metabolic rates for normal subjects 78 years of age was on the average 26% less than those at age 18. This latter research, however, also revealed that the 26% alteration was of the same order as the variance among subjects of any age; in other words, some normal subjects at age 18 could have a cerebral metabolic rate for glucose 26% less than other normal 18-year-olds (Kuhl, Metter, Riege, & Hawkins, 1985). When PET and CT scan changes in normal elderly subjects have been compared, data have shown that changes can occur in the latter without any in the former—again suggesting that, up to a point, structural losses do not necessarily result in concomitant metabolic deficits (de Leon, George, & Ferris, 1986).

PET findings have been more significant in comparisons between normal aging subjects and those with Alzheimer's disease. With the progression of Alzheimer's disease, reductions in glucose metabolism become more pronounced. Moreover, PET scan changes with advancing Alzheimer's disease have been more marked than CT scan changes. This suggests that PET is potentially more useful than CT in the diagnosis of Alzheimer's disease. It is not apparent, however, how early in the progression of Alzheimer's disease that implicating PET changes occur; it is, of course, in the early stage of the disorder where diagnosis is most difficult (Riege & Metter, 1988).

Divergent structural and metabolic findings are significant in their potential relevance to brain plasticity. If mild to moderate structural changes can occur (e.g., if there can be mild to moderate brain tissue loss) without clinically important metabolic consequences, then the clinical deficits associated with marked structural impairment could be potentially mitigated by neurochemical means (e.g., by drugs). Similarly, to the extent that disorder in the aging brain has more of a physiologic basis than a structural one, metabolic or pharmacologic interventions might effect significant clinical improvement. This is a hope with Alzheimer's disease.

Paradoxical Turns Toward Normality in Aging

Health and illness are not only concepts of relative states, they exhibit flux independent of age. Many diseases, for example, are commonly characterized by alternating periods of flare-ups and remissions. Occasionally, too, seemingly paradoxical effects can be observed where the same changes in one individual that could result in the development of new clinical symptoms, could in another individual bring about reduction in certain pathological conditions. Consider the aging eye. As one grows older there is a loss of efficiency in focusing vision at different distances, due to changes in the lens of the eye. This loss of accommodation with age is known as *presbyopia.* Remarkably, individuals who were near-sighted (myopic) prior to the development of presbyopia may, for the first time in years, be able to read without glasses, with the onset of presbyopia. These individuals experience the phenomenon of their eyesight improving with age, as a result of counterbalancing lens pathology; the lens, which was originally pathologically bent causing nearsightedness, begins to bend in the opposite direction, thereby alleviating the myopia (Newell, 1982).

A related phenomenon has been hypothesized in the "burnout" of schizophrenia. As mentioned above, an excess of dopamine is associated with psychotic states and with schizophrenia in particular. Many of the drugs used to treat schizophrenia have mechanisms of action that block the neurotransmission of dopamine. There are estimates of 30 to 40% of schizophrenics experiencing a gradual reduction ("burnout") of the intensity of their symptoms with advancing years, even in the absence of drug therapy. An hypothesis holds that according to the dopamine-excess view of schizophrenia, symptomatic individuals who had relatively high dopamine levels would then, due to the loss of dopamine-producing neurons with aging, gradually return toward a more normal state of functioning (Finch, 1985a).

A further example can be seen with sexual changes in the aging male. The latency period prior to orgasm in aging men is prolonged. Whereas for some this may be experienced as a delay in their orgasm, others view it as increased orgasmic control. Due to this change, older men who had suffered through their earlier years with premature ejaculation may find themselves developing an orgasmic pattern that approaches that of normal younger males (Davidson, 1985).

These observations about normality, schizophrenia, and aging once again illustrate the potentially enormous relevance of studying health and illness in later life as a source for fundamental new insights about the prevention and treatment of disorders independent of age. Thus, by studying the natural physiologic changes in the aging brain that operate to mitigate schizophrenia in later life, one might gain new understanding about preventing or better treating schizophrenia in earlier adulthood. We can see how research on the aging brain offers an important new window for peering into the mysteries of the world of neuroscience, and a new door perhaps for gaining access to clues for therapeutic breakthroughs relevant to the old and young alike.

Memory and Aging

Memory remains an elusive phenomenon, hard to pin down as to how and where in the brain it is stored. Views vary and overlap (Squire & Butters, 1984). There are those who portray each neuron as having a key role in memory formation and storage, with memory traces being incorporated into enduring protein components of the nerve cell (Restak, 1980). This view could be consistent with the lack of replication of neurons once they are formed early in life. At birth, the vast majority of neurons have already been formed, while by age two the human brain approaches its adult size, weight, and number of cells. Why new neurons do not develop in the brain beyond the first few years of life is not clear, and invites speculation. If cortical nerve cells were to replicate further as one grew older, might this make the information storage network chaotic, since stability and consistency of structural stores of memory would appear to be required for efficient retrieval and synthesis of ideas? In other words, if new neurons were to replace existing ones, might this result in earlier memories being lost with the replaced nerve cells; if new neurons were to supplement existing ones, might this result in a situation analogous to new memories being recorded on blank tapes as opposed to building upon existing ones for greater synchrony?

Others portray memory as residing less in neurons than in relationships between neurons (Fuster, 1984). This second view, which is not incompatible with storage functions on the part of individual nerve cells, suggests that memory resides in a contingent of neurons only as much and as firmly as they are interconnected—this being accomplished through the elaborate circuitry of intercommunicating *dendrites* (see Figure 2.3). Thus memory would be as widely distributed over the cerebral cortex as are the cells in the network for that memory. Fuster (1984) suggests that a given cell or group of cells may be part of many such networks (or distributed systems of associations) and, therefore, of many memories. Different parts of the brain through which these networks pass assume functions in addition to adding neurons to the circuitry. Different brain locations also function as associative centers where memories and thoughts are integrated and interpreted (see Figure 2.2).

Studies of memory in the aging brain benefit as much from behavioral techniques as high technology (Poon, 1986). Indeed observations about an individual's behavior often point to regions of the brain where high tech imaging should probe in search of neural explanations for different memory patterns.

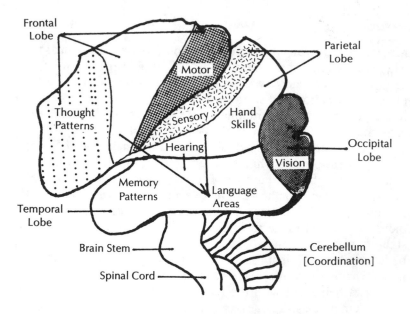

Figure 2.2 Side view of brain's surface from front (*left*) to back (*right*) illustrating functional and association areas. The cerebral cortex of the brain, which governs memory processes and higher intellectual activities, consists mainly of the surface gray cell layers of the frontal, parietal, temporal, and occipital lobes, in addition to the hippocampus which has an important role in memory functioning and is formed by an infolding of the lower surface of the temporal lobe.

To illustrate, in examining certain perceived decrements in memory performance with aging, behavioral observations have led to causative factors being portrayed in terms of "inefficient" functioning rather than clear breakage or loss of component structures in the central nervous system. The fact that changes in the way an older person's memory is challenged can improve the efficiency of recall—to the level of accuracy of a younger adult—supports this view. The following example has been given: Some older people might have considerable difficulty in describing a route through city streets, although these same individuals can find their own way perfectly well when actually on these streets. In the latter situation, the "context" provides "support and guidance" with respect to each successive turn and decision en route (Craik, 1984); that the context restores recall demonstrates that the original memory is still there and provides further evidence of the potential for memory plasticity in the aging brain.

Here, too, research on aging offers new insights into processes fundamental to all age groups. Aging brain research offers new insights and hypotheses about the nature of memory and associated cognitive phenomena across the life cycle. For example, comparing affected neurons from those with Alzheimer's disease (where memory is impaired) with normal nerve cells from healthy aging brains (where memory is intact) may lead to more specifics about the nature of memory processes. In Figure 2.3, which depicts two neurons under electron microscopic magnification, the neurofibers are of interest.

Neurofibers comprise thin fibrils, protein in composition, located more within the axons (an axis cylinder of a neuron that conducts impulses away from the cell body of the neuron) than the cell bodies and dendrites of neurons (Iqbal, Grundke-Iqbal, Wisniewski, & Terry, 1978). The func-

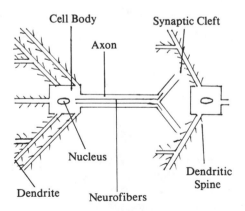

Figure 2.3 Two neurons magnified under an electron microscope. × 100,000.

tions of neurofibers are not known, though they have been implicated in varied physiologic events, including the induction of impulses within the nerve cell. The different types of neurofibers in the normal aging neuron have characteristic widths and shapes. In Alzheimer's disease, fibrils of different widths and shapes from normal ones are seen within large numbers of neurons in the cerebral cortex. There has been a debate about the neurofibrils in Alzheimer's disease (referred to as neurofibrillary *tangles* because of their twisted, helical shape) as to whether they simply represent anatomical disfigurations of normal fibrils, or whether they are aberrant structures with an abnormal protein composition as well. Normal fibrils that become tangled might be compared with telephone wires becoming knotted and thereby interfering with clear communication; aberrant fibrils being produced within the axon could be analogous to segments of string being patched into wire, with scrambled communication resulting. Given theories about memory functioning that address both the role of intraneuronal protein and the nature of intercommunication between neurons, the neurofibrillary tangles in Alzheimer's disease could effect disturbances in both of these mechanisms. Further research on both the normal aging brain and on Alzheimer's disease will undoubtedly provide new insights into the nature of memory and intellectual functioning. Through this focus on the aging brain and its most dread illness, scientists are likely to expand their fundamental understanding of cognitive processes that are part of the fabric of the human condition across the entire life cycle.

3

Behavior and the Aging Brain

Behavioral considerations broadly encompass intellectual functioning, mood, personality, and behavior.

INTELLECTUAL CAPACITY WITH AGING

Perhaps no area in aging has elicited more concern than that of intellectual functioning. Both stereotypes and misinformation have been particularly strong here. What does the scientific literature reveal about normal intellectual functioning with aging (Shock, Greulich, Andres, et al., 1984)? In 1961 Owens reported on a longitudinal study of cognitive performance in 96 men, average age 61, who had originally been tested in 1919 as freshmen at Iowa State University (Owens, 1966). The key finding of this study was that on the average there was little change in intellectual test scores as these men aged from 50 to 60. A report by Owens in 1953 showed increments in verbal ability and total score of intellectual performance with these men as they moved from age 20 to age 50, though numerical ability showed a slight decline (Owens, 1953). These studies were among the first to raise serious doubts about the presumed normal decline in mental abilities with advancing age that had been inferred from earlier cross-sectional research.

Unlike *longitudinal* investigations, which compare performances of the same individual at different ages, *cross-sectional* studies compare performances of different individuals in different age groups where it is very difficult to control for such factors as common educational background, emotional development, and other cultural, historical, and environmental influences. In other words, if a cross-sectional study had been carried out in 1970 comparing 20-year-olds with 70-year-olds, the fact that one group had been educated in pre-Sputnik days and the other during the space race would undoubtedly have had a skewing effect on the results. On the other hand, a longitudinal study comparing the results of the 20-year-olds with their own performances 50 years later, when they are 70, is likely to provide more accurate data about the impact of aging on various performance measures.

In 1955, a 12-year longitudinal study of men, median age 71, was initiated at the National Institute of Mental Health (Birren, Butler, Greenhouse, Sokoloff & Yarrow, 1974). The goal of the study was to examine a broad range of variables in individuals of advanced age in whom disease was absent or minimal; the study aimed particularly *to separate the impact of aging from that of illness.* Of note in these healthy aging subjects as they moved on the average from their 70s to their 80s was that while certain intellectual functions declined, others improved. Declines were noted in the speed of carrying out different tasks, in the quality of sentence completions, and in the quality of a test known as Draw-a-Person (in this "graphomotor" test the subject is instructed to "draw a picture of a person, the best one you can, make it a whole person"; it provides, through the analysis of perceptual and motor skills, information on intellectual performance and whether brain damage might be present). On the other hand, vocabulary improved as did picture arrangement; this was shown in the improved results from the respective subtests on vocabulary and picture arrangement within the Wechsler Adult Intelligence Scale (WAIS). In terms of everyday life, this suggests that certain activities requiring quick reactions or a high degree of precision might not be carried out as well by older adults in general, though the ability to understand one's situation and learn from new experiences is maintained in later life.

Moreover, certain age associated declines can be misleading if examined out of context, as in the case of speed of response. A study comparing speed and *accuracy* of response between young and old (66 to 83 years of age) subjects found that when the elderly *took enough time,* no significant difference in accuracy occurred among the different age groups (Sharps & Gollin, 1987).

Tests were also carried out to measure IQ over an 11-year period. Despite the limitations of IQ tests in general, the results are fascinating. At the start of the study in 1956, when the healthy subjects were generally in their 70s, IQs averaged 108; six years later, IQs averaged 100; eleven years from the start, healthy subjects, now generally in their 80s, had an average IQ of 110 (Granick & Patterson, 1971). Hence, with the maintenance of overall health, there was no statistical change in overall IQ performance with these individuals. Where decrements did occur, the influence of illness was implicated—not aging per se. More specifically, decrements in intellectual performance with advancing age were found to be significantly greater in subjects who had developed cardiovascular disease than in those who remained healthy. The linkage of cardiovascular illness to intellectual impairment was described in a later study as well, where more frequent memory problems were found to be associated with heart disease (Barrett & Watkins, 1986). The point is not that one fails to witness cognitive decline in the age group of the elderly; clearly many older adults do exhibit such changes. Rather, the point is that *the nature, inevitability, prevalence, and cause of such declines in later life all have come under question.*

The National Institute of Mental Health longitudinal aging study made an important contribution by illustrating the impact of illness on intellectual functioning with aging, while showing how relative stability in overall intellectual capacities could continue into advanced old age in those who maintained good general health (Granick & Patterson, 1971). The role of disorder (not normal aging) as a cause of significant cognitive dysfunction in later life was becoming clear. No longer could noticeable intellectual decline in later life be dismissed as just the inevitable consequence of growing old. These findings challenged the clinician to look at significant impairments in later life as symptoms of potentially modifiable disease as opposed to manifestations of the relentless destiny of advancing years. The stage was set for the search for treatments and effective clinical interventions to modify brain disease in the elderly—to modify the intellectual and behavioral dysfunction that accompanies organic mental disorders in older adults. The dramatic new attention to Alzheimer's disease highlights this new awareness.

The findings of stable overall intellectual functioning in later life are being replicated in different ways in an increasing number of studies. More and more they point to the conclusion that many elderly individuals continue to score at the level of middle-aged adults on cognitive tests. "In other words, for significant portions of the elderly population, intellectual decline cannot be demonstrated" (Stagner, 1985). In fact, one of the most stable elements in the aging mind is reasoning ability. A study by Schaie, following individuals into their 80s, detected no reliable decrement in reasoning ability at any age among those he studied (Schaie & Parham, 1977).

Some of this research examines the question of intellectual stability over time not with psychometric tests, but by measuring performance in real-world terms; studies in the workplace evaluating job performance, for instance, fit into this category. Kelleher and Quirk (1973) analyzed the productivity of 6,000 clerical workers from U.S. Department of Labor data and found no significant difference by age in terms of total output. Moreover, older workers were found to be steadier than younger ones and equal to them in accuracy. Job satisfaction has also been described as another plus with aging. A survey by the Opinion Research Corporation found an increase in job satisfaction with increasing age among managers, clerks, and hourly employees alike (Stagner, 1985).

While one line of research examines the areas where capacity is maintained with aging, another pursues the question of whether any skills *improve.* Clay (1956), in a study of proofreaders, found that as a group those over 60 performed better than younger workers. Dennis (1966) explored productivity in relation to creativity by studying the bibliographies of scholars between 20 and 80 years of age. He discovered that scholars were as prolific in their 70s as in their 40s, and were actually more so in their 60s. An illustration of the tendency to trivialize the maintenance of talent with aging is suggested by the observations of Kogan (1975) who points out that individuals making discoveries early in their careers and then continuing their work in that area might no longer be seen as creative, despite maintaining the same quality in their productivity. Thus if one's seminal achievement occurs earlier in life, and the years that follow focus on the further development of the breakthrough, the latter years are often dismissed as *derivative,* even though they might result in greater maturity or application of one's attainment. Creativity in later life will be reviewed in considerable detail in Chapter 9.

In a detailed review of studies on intelligence and problem solving among the aging, Schaie (1980) concludes with the following perspective:

> I would like to caution clinicians once again that most of what we know about intelligence and problem solving in the elderly has been learned using instruments and techniques developed for children and young adults. We are only at the beginning of charting adult functioning with techniques which are truly indigenous to the elderly. It is quite possible, therefore, that what appears as disadvantage when compared with the young, may simply represent a regrouping and re-expression of function which might be quite appropriate and adaptive for the old. Research now in progress in a number of laboratories will hopefully shed light on this major issue. (p. 280)

LEARNING CAPACITY AND AGING

The capacity to learn knows no endpoint in the human life cycle. The findings, alluded to above, of continued growth of vocabulary among many individuals well into advanced old age support this statement. In my own study of mentally healthy older adults between the ages of 65 and 102, examples of new intellectual growth and inquiry are abundant. One of these subjects, an 82-year-old woman with a high school education, had only since her late 70s developed an interest in reading books. This interest, however, so motivated her that in the six months prior to my first interview with her she had devoured 21 novels.

The lessons from widows in my study have been equally revealing. Many of these older women had gone through their marriages in the so-called traditional pre-women's liberation mode, where a disproportionate amount of household management was carried out by their husbands. A significant number of the wives became emotionally vulnerable because of the high degree of dependency that developed. Following the deaths of their spouses, many of these women found themselves for the first time in the position of having to manage everything from checkbooks to circuit breakers. Not only do many women in this new situation eventually master their new challenges but they also commonly experience a sense of exhilaration in the discovery of latent skills and abilities for independence.

Recognition of ongoing learning capacity in later life has been blurred by negative stereotypes like "you can't teach an old dog new tricks." In actuality, this pejorative equating of older persons with dogs is not even accurate about our canine companions; at quite an old age, dogs can indeed be taught new tricks (Berwick, 1983). And so can humans. A study on "the effects of videogame playing on the response selection processing of elderly adults" found that a seven-week training program using videogames improved both (1) the *speed* of response and (2) the *accuracy* of making a particular selection in elderly subjects (Clark, Lanphear, & Riddick, 1987). Perhaps the paradigm in general for this age group as to the capacity for new tricks is the story of Harland Sanders (a.k.a. Colonel Sanders) who tried something new and made a fortune after the age of 65. It was at the age of 74 that the Kentucky Colonel sold his secret recipe for "finger lickin' good chicken" and made his millions, remaining in the limelight even as a nonagenarian (Britannica, 1985e).

Moreover, learning capacity needs to be examined not only in intellectual terms, but in emotional and life experience parameters as well. The admonition to "do it until you get it right" acknowledges the involvement of time if not age in the learning process. Poon (1987, p. 380) summarizes the scientific literature on this topic by pointing out that "when a number of variables associated with a learning task are taken into account, the chronological age of the learner has not been shown to provide a significant amount of influence on performance." Willis (1985, p. 843) reached the same conclusion: "The research literature in adult developmental psychology demonstrates that older adults have a substantial learning potential and presents evidence of a special need for continuing educational opportunities in later life."

Among the major variables that adversely affect learning in later life are, again, poor health and psychological turmoil. At the same time, the impact of clinical interventions in such cases further illustrates learning potential by demonstrating the capacity of the elderly to develop new coping strategies in the face of emotional conflict (Gatz, Popkin, Pino, & VandenBos, 1985); this will be reflected in considerably greater detail in the discussion on psychotherapy with older adults in Chapter 4.

Moving from the scientific literature to that of the arts, we find similar lessons poignantly portrayed. One of the classic literary works that is a powerful treatment of this theme—to learn, to develop new strategies, to change—is Charles Dickens's *Christmas Carol*. The emotional liberation of the aged Scrooge wonderfully portrays the enduring human capacity to face crises and grow, to break out of ruts, to learn from mistakes—to finally get it right. In a poignant transition Scrooge exclaims, "I will live in the Past, Present, and the Future. The spirits of all Three shall strive within me. I will not shut out the lessons they teach" (Dickens, 1984).

A similar theme is dramatically dealt with in *Wild Strawberries,* the film masterpiece on old age by the Swedish writer-director Ingmar Bergman. Erikson Erikson in his lectures on stages of the human life cycle shows *Wild Strawberries* to illustrate the tension between opportunities and obstacles to achieving the ultimate "maturity, wisdom, and integrity" that can come to the elderly. Erikson (1963) then translates this ultimate learning for the aged into a life cycle lesson for the young when he describes the relation of older adult integrity to infantile trust, suggesting that "healthy children will not fear life if their elders have integrity enough not to fear death."

BEHAVIORAL TRAITS IN LATER LIFE: CAUTIOUSNESS AND RISK-TAKING

Moving from stereotypes about intellectual and learning capacities in later life, one finds comparable mythology and misunderstanding about behavioral and personality traits in older adults. Consider the issue of caution and the elderly, where research is interesting. A study by Okun and Elias (1977) showed that older individuals *were* more cautious than younger adults about risk-taking *in situations where the payoff was predictable and at a constant level.* If the size of the payoff depended on the degree of risk, however, then the elderly were *not* more cautious than younger individuals. Otherwise, one would not see so many older adults at the one-armed bandits of Atlantic City. The Okun results imply that with aging one may develop better judgment about when risk-taking is likely to have a greater payoff.

An example of the need to differentiate illness in later life from the normal concomitants of the aging process can also be observed here.

Specifically, it has been found that anxiety can result in cautiousness which in turn delays decision-making processes and reactions (Thomae, 1980). Excessive cautiousness in the elderly, in other words, may signal underlying anxiety or a related clinical disorder. In a related sense, an older person, who because of frailty or disability is more vulnerable or less mobile, *should* be more careful in approaching life in general. The difference in concepts here lies in distinguishing an increase in carefulness as an appropriate, adaptive response to the demands of reality from a maladaptive overcautiousness resulting from inner fears.

PERSONALITY AND AGING: DISPOSITIONS AND DEVELOPMENT

A major stereotype about the effect of aging on personality is that older persons tend to experience an exaggeration of earlier forms of behavior—particularly their less desirable qualities. This view is expressed in comments like "the elderly become more like themselves with aging." Hence, if a person were stingy in his/her youth, by old age he/she would be an outright miser—the image of Scrooge. Research finds that when certain responses grow increasingly exaggerated, maladaptive, and unmodifiable over time, neurosis rather than normal aging may be to blame (Bergmann, 1978).

Several theories of psychological development with aging describe behavioral change, flexibility, and capacity for growth as one accumulates years (Siegler, 1980). Jung, for example, theorizes a fundamental change in the direction of one's psychological orientation in the second half of the life cycle. He offers the analogy that "after having lavished its light upon the world, the sun withdraws its rays in order to illuminate itself" (Campbell, 1972). This view is similar to that of others who see the transition from midlife to old age as one characterized by a change in orientation from external issues and a focus on work to an emphasis on internal feelings and interpersonal relationships (Siegler, 1980). Jung (in Campbell, 1972) theorizes further, with his mixed psychological and poetic style, that:

We cannot live in the afternoon of life according to the programme of life's morning; for what was great in the morning will be little at evening, and what in the morning was true will at evening have become a lie. . . A human being would certainly not grow to be seventy or eighty years old if this longevity had no meaning for the species. The afternoon of human life must also have a significance of its own and cannot be merely a pitiful appendage to life's morning. The significance of the morning undoubtedly lies in the development of the individual, our entrenchment in the outer world, the propagation of our kind, and the care of our children. This is the obvious purpose of nature. But when this purpose has been attained—and more than attained—shall the earning of money, the extension of conquests, and the expansion of life go steadily on beyond the bounds of all reason and sense? Whoever carries over into the afternoon the law of the morning, or the natural aim, must pay for it with damage to his soul, just as surely as a growing youth who tries to carry over his childish egoism into adult life must pay for this mistake with social failure. Money-making, social achievement, family and posterity are nothing but plain nature, not culture. Culture lies outside the purpose of nature. Could by any chance culture be the meaning and purpose of the second half of life? (p. 17)

Erikson, too, depicts different tasks at different stages of life, describing eight distinct development milestones, each one confronting the individual with a specific challenge or crisis to surmount. For example, Erikson theorizes that the baby struggles to achieve a sense of basic trust versus mistrust, that the young adult struggles to achieve intimacy as opposed to isolation, that the older adult struggles to achieve ego integrity over despair or disdain (Erikson, 1963). Common to these stage theories of psychological development is the concept of emerging new life issues, rather than stereotypic regression into earlier behavioral modes.

Whereas a pathologic response to stress can induce regression in the elderly, as it can in any age group, normal responses to stress or threats often differ with older adults as compared to younger ones. In the Baltimore Longitudinal Study of Aging (begun in 1958), 28 different coping mechanisms were examined in response to stress among different age groups. The most frequently used coping mechanisms in response to stress across age groups were "restraint, rational action, expression of feelings, and positive thinking"; the least frequently used were "self-blame, intellectual denial, passivity, sedation, and hostile reaction" (Shock, et al., 1984).

Moreover, older people (aged 50–64 and 65–89) were less likely than younger ones (aged 21–49) to use hostile reaction and escapist fantasy. These findings tend to contradict the notion that older individuals are prone to the use of primitive and immature defenses, which represent variants on the "more like themselves" theme. It was concluded that "older men and women do not rigidly maintain habits of coping that, although appropriate in youth, have outlived their usefulness. Instead, as stresses change, so do coping responses" (Shock, et al., 1984).

All of this is not to say that one's basic personality changes with aging (Costa et al., 1987). The point is that behavioral and psychological adaptiveness continues with aging, and does not, under normal circumstances, give way to regression or rigidity in personality traits (Thomae, 1980). Indeed a number of studies find no increase in behavioral rigidity with aging (Thomae, 1980). Where comparisons portray older adults as appearing more rigid than younger individuals, cohort differences (generational differences as a factor of having been brought up during different historical periods)—and not age differences—are more likely being described.

Examples of behavioral and attitudinal flexibility in my own study of the mentally healthy elderly are ever present. With many, it is as if retirement is more like a curtain between acts; scenes change, and the characters continue to evolve. Sometimes a different approach to a situation may seem simple on the surface, but can represent high emotional drama and significant inner development. Such was the sense I got from the following episode described by a 76-year-old woman I interviewed. She was telling me about a trip she took to Italy a year earlier. At one point in her recounting, she recalled a specific occurrence in the airport at Rome. Before she proceeded very far in the narrative, she paused to inquire as to whether she was boring me with dull details. I remarked that sometimes seemingly mundane experiences offer us glimpses of bigger issues in life. She resumed, explaining that while in Italy she learned that a very dear friend back home had died. She wanted very much to attend the funeral, which necessitated an immediate return, much earlier than had been planned. This in turn meant that she would have to go directly to the airport to get a new ticket and catch the first available flight. Time was of the essence. She arrived at the airport 30 minutes before flight time, and found a long line at the counter for purchasing new tickets. She went to the end of the line. Time was passing quickly; the line moved slowly. She thought that she would never get the ticket in time and would thus miss the flight and the funeral. Mobilizing her courage, she acted in a way she never had before during more than seven decades. She cut in line—for the first time in her life. Despite excusing herself, the language barrier prevented adequate explanation to others in line. She felt fortunate, though, that her inability to understand Italian prevented her from comprehending the expletives that were hurled at her. Her pulse was pumping, but she kept her poise and her new position in line, miraculously obtaining the ticket and getting on the plane just in the nick of time. It had been no small step for her to do this. In retrospect she realized that her risk-taking and success had left her physically exhausted but emotionally exhilarated. Only in looking back at that episode did she realize that a turning point had occurred in how she had been approaching challenging situations since then; she realized she had become more assertive and persistent. "Not bad for approaching 80," we both agreed. Rather than causing a regression to an earlier stage of behavior—or acting more like themselves—normal aging for many means discovering new aspects of themselves.

SELF-IMAGE AND AGING

It is not uncommon to think that the aging mind becomes increasingly beleaguered with dread and despair. But according to the 1974 national survey by Harris and Associates for the National Council on Aging, the findings reflected something quite different (Harris & Associates, 1975). The survey, sampling more than 4,000 persons (including approximately 2,600 aged 65 and older), elicited reactions to both positive and negative statements. The section on life satisfaction is particularly interesting. Those 65 and older were compared to those 18–64 years of age. Some of the statements and responses follow:

Positive Statements

I've gotten pretty much what I expected out of life.

> More of those aged 65+ (a high 82%) felt that this statement was true for them than did those aged 18–64 (80%).

As I look back on my life, I am fairly well satisfied.

> More of those aged 65+ (a high 87%) felt that the statement was true for them than did those aged 18–64 (85%).

I would not change my past life even if I could.

> More of those aged 65+ (62%) felt that this statement was true for them than did those aged 18–64 (56%).

Negative Statements

Most of the things I do are boring or monotonous.

> Only 14% of those aged 65+ felt that this statement was true for them, as compared to a similar percentage (12%) of those aged 18–64 who felt this way.

Compared to other people, I get down in the dumps too often.

> Only 13% of those aged 65+ felt that this statement was true for them, as compared to a similar percentage (14%) of those aged 18–64 who felt this way.

My life could be happier than it is now.

While 45% of those aged 65+ felt this statement was true for them, an even greater percentage (49%) of those aged 18–64 felt the same way.

In addition to the above positive feelings on the part of the elderly, and taking into account these areas where negativism is low, approximately three out of four elderly individuals surveyed felt that "the things I do are as interesting to me as they ever were." In addition, over half were making plans for and expressing positive expectations about the future. It is not that the survey was without areas where the elderly were less positive or more negative than younger adults. Rather, what was remarkable was the number of areas where the elderly compared very favorably or even better than other age groups.

In another study on quality of life in relation to age, done by the American Institutes of Research, one thousand 50-year-olds and one thousand 70-year-olds were interviewed. Only slight differences were reported between these two age groups with regard to overall quality of their lives, with about 85% indicating that the quality of their lives was "good, very good, or excellent" (Birren & Renner, 1980).

CONCEPT OF DEATH AND AGING

To what extent do thoughts of death weigh heavily on the aging mind? Here, too, research findings diverge from popular views (Kastenbaum, 1985; Reker, Peacock, & Wong, 1987). Research shows that while thoughts about death are more on the minds of older persons, dread of death is less prevalent in the elderly as compared to other age groups (Kalish, 1976). To be thinking or talking more about death is not the same as fearing or dreading it. It is not surprising that ideas or conversations about death are more common among the elderly. After all, older people are more likely to have peers and older relatives who have died or are dying.

Even the reading of obituaries by the elderly is often misunderstood by younger persons, who see it as an obsessive preoccupation with death. Many older people, however, point out that they have too often been embarrassed by *not* learning about the death of an old colleague or acquaintance until some time after the funeral, and thus not having been able to pay their respects at the proper time. An older person is simply more likely to have an acquaintance listed in the obituaries than is a younger adult.

To understand dread of death, one has to examine its context. Dread of death in later life indeed seems to be most uncommon in an older person who *is not dying or is not experiencing some major loss at the time.* It is the presence of a terminal illness, an underlying depression, or other emotional conflict—not the awareness of aging in itself—that predisposes to death anxiety in certain elderly individuals. Interestingly, dread of death as a normal phenomenon has been described as typically more common in middle age than in later life (Kalish, 1976). It is in middle age when one takes a critical turn in thinking for the first time about how much time is left, as opposed to how much has gone by. Once people begin to think more deeply about their time remaining, they find themselves confronting an existential awareness of their own mortality. When this *first* occurs, reactive feelings can be profound. Angst can swell in the individual—dread about what will ultimately follow. By later life, however, perspective is restored. Those who are aging well have adjusted to their altered time frame, and denial as a normal psychological defense mechanism when experienced in the right proportions once again sets in constructively; the right amount of denial facilitates a constructive repression or control of one's awareness of always moving chronologically closer to death. This is the same denial of our fundamental mortality that has allowed explorers to climb the highest mountains and the astronauts to go to the moon. Too much denial is, of course, maladaptive; it can make one reckless or else result in varied psychological disturbances. Denial in the proper amount facilitates the daring necessary for great achievement; it is also required to help one focus much more on life than on death, to live well each day.

It is a different matter, though, when one has a terminal illness or is suffering from depression. A terminal illness brings an awareness of dying that breaks through denial and can lead to despondency. Here, too, the majority eventually come to terms with their fate and develop a reasonable acceptance of their condition (Brown, Henteleff, Barakat, & Rowe, 1986). But the healthy older individual is no more dying than a younger adult in good health, and as life expectancy statistics apply to aggregates and not individuals, there is little reason for most elderly persons to feel that death is imminent. After all, at age 65, a given individual could well live another two decades, if not two generations; more and more are.

The situation with depression is similar. At any age, depression clouds one's thinking. A depressed state increases the likelihood of thoughts about death. It is commonly remarked that the thoughts of a depressed young man make him sound like an old man. It would be more accurate to say that the thoughts of a depressed young man have much in common with those of a depressed old man. A major precipitator of depression in any age group is loss. The elderly are at increased risk of loss, though they are better prepared for certain types of loss than younger people.

This better preparation may be a factor of certain losses being generally perceived as at higher risk with aging—more expected or "on-time" in later life—and, as a corollary, unexpected or untimely in earlier adulthood (Hagestad & Neugarten, 1985; Neugarten, Moore, & Lowe, 1965). Disability, for example, though neither a normal nor inevitable part of aging per se, is more anticipated in later life. Nonetheless, loss at any stage of the life cycle can seriously disrupt emotional equilibrium, and, if great enough, lead to depression. Loss comes in many forms—loss of spouse, loss of physical health, loss of economic security, loss of self-esteem, and so forth.

There is important clinical significance to this discussion. When an elderly individual seems preoccupied with thoughts of death, it may be doing the person a serious disservice to dismiss these concerns by offering false reassurances that it is normal to feel this way. It is highly likely that this older person is not ruminating about death simply because existential thoughts have come to mind that the time to die is coming closer. Rather, the individual is much more likely to be troubled by emotional conflict. Perhaps a son or daughter is going through a messy divorce, and the older individual experiences feelings of unfounded guilt about being a failure as a parent, as if he or she had somehow done something wrong in bringing up the child. Self-esteem suffers, depression may result, and with it increased preoccupation with dying. Distressing thoughts about death, particularly persisting ones, should be regarded as signals of underlying disorder with the elderly—not as a normal concomitant of aging.

RETIREMENT AND AGING

There are competing points of view about retirement, one group emphasizes its negative consequences for psychological adjustment, health, and mortality, while another paints it as a welcome relief from an unrewarding, arduous, and emotionally trying life of work (Ekerdt, 1987; Robinson, Coberly, & Paul, 1985; Sheppard, 1976). Still others see it as an opportunity to achieve more independence and to pursue long desired interests previously crowded out by the everyday demands of a work schedule.

There is a body of literature that stresses the relationship between retirement and loss of social status and self-esteem. Other investigators have challenged such assumptions, describing the circumstances under which retirement occurs as determining how well one will do after retiring. Streib's findings (1971), for example, point to *prior attitudes and expectations* as the most important predictor of adjustment to retirement; thus, a positive orientation toward retirement is seen as likely to be met with a positive post-retirement experience.

Good health at the time of retirement is viewed by other researchers to be a positive predictor for future life satisfaction. Poor health, on the other hand, often forces premature retirement for many. Those retiring for health reasons, who in their minds are not ready to retire, appear to be more vulnerable to difficulty in adjusting to leaving the preferred milieu of work (Parnes & Nestel, 1981). Poor health continuing into retirement or beginning during that period obviously in itself colors the retirement experience for affected individuals. The poor health group represents a subset of a larger group whose retirement is seen as involuntary or compulsory. To leave the work place involuntarily is believed to raise the risk of retirement having a negative impact (Jaffe, 1972).

Another viewpoint concerning health problems around retirement time is also apposite here. Morbidity and mortality rates in the postretirement period may be misleading in that poor health, rather than being a consequence of retirement, is often its cause. In a study of 500 men and women aged 67 or less who had retired *in good health* and were evaluated within three years of retiring, reports of their health status were striking (Sheldon, McEwan, & Ryser, 1975). Upon being asked whether there had been any change in their health since retirement, 65.5% reported no change; 10.4% indicated a change for the worse; remarkably, 24.1% described a change for the better. Hence, nearly 90% had stayed the same or even improved. Tentative explanations by the investigators for the large percentage who either maintained or bettered their health were that these individuals, because of their age, were more conscientious about tending to their health needs, and because they were retired had more time to seek proper medical attention. In my study of the mentally healthy elderly, a number of individuals have been identified who have experienced a subsiding of various stress-related physical health problems since retiring. For these people it appears that the pressures of the workplace caused somatic problems ranging from gastrointestinal upset to an aggravation of angina. Leaving this stressfilled environment led to an alleviation of symptoms in many who had suffered such problems.

In addition to the role of one's attitude toward retirement, readiness for it, and decision-forcing events like illness, other factors influence one's orientation to it. The nature of one's work also can play an important part. As one reaches "retirement age," whether one's job is satisfying or dissatisfying takes on understandable importance. A worker on an assembly line who has performed the same demanding routine for years might be looking forward to retirement much more than a top administrator who faces challenges and rewards.

Not to be overlooked is one of the major determinants in both the decision to retire and the quality of retirement—namely, *finances!* If one does not anticipate having adequate resources to maintain a reasonable post-retirement standard of living, then one's attitude toward retiring is likely mixed at best, and the freedom to enjoy retirement could well be compromised.

In my own study of mental health issues and the elderly in general, if physical health and finances are not problems, then a key factor that appears to influence the quality of retirement living is the social portfolio of interests, activities, and interpersonal relationships that one brings into or else plans to develop while being retired. Those well prepared in this regard seem to enjoy and do well in retirement; those poorly prepared in these ways appear more at risk for trouble. There are those, too, who use the technique of partial retirement as an approach to bridging these two worlds.

To a large extent, the enormous growth of the elderly population has changed the context and meaning of retirement. Rather than being looked at primarily as the process of departing from the work force, retirement has increasingly come to represent a new stage in the life cycle (Ekerdt, 1987). The focus on retirement has expanded and shifted—evolving from concerns about adapting to a loss or change of identity vis-à-vis the work place to anticipation of new life experiences facilitated by increased time for leisure, grandparenting, and exploring new lifestyle opportunities. As a result, individual and societal planning for retirement living have increased, adding to the probability and frequency of well-being during this new life phase.

ACTIVITY AND AGING

Confronting yet another myth about aging, the 1974 national survey by Harris and Associates found remarkable similarity in activity patterns in comparing those aged 65 and older to individuals aged 18–64; the following findings have been extracted (Louis Harris & Associates, 1975, p. 57):

> The interesting finding is that the older public seems no more or less likely to spend "a lot of time" on most of the pastimes tested than those under 65. Comparable numbers of the old and the young, for example, said that they spend a lot of time "sleeping" (16% of those 65+ vs. 15% of those 18–64 reported spending a lot of time sleeping), "reading" (36% of those 65+ vs. 38% of those 18–64), "participating in fraternal or community organizations" (17% of those 65+ vs. 13% of those 18–64), "going for walks" (25% of those 65+ vs. 22% of those 18–64), etc.
>
> In three areas, those under 65 are much more likely than the older public to spend a lot of time: in caring for younger or older members of the family, in working part time or full time, and in participating in sports. The public 65 and older, on the other hand, is more likely to spend a lot of time watching television than is the younger public. But apart from these four areas, the involvement of

the young and the old in the activities mentioned was nearly comparable. Even with watching television, the difference was not so great (36% of those 65+ vs. 23% of those 18–64 reported spending a lot of time), while in other passive activities more time was spent by those under 65 than by the older group (37% of those 18–64 reported spending a lot of time sitting and thinking as compared to only 31% of those 65+).

These findings lend support to the *activity theory* as opposed to the *disengagement theory* in explaining the social phenomenology of successful aging. The *disengagement theory* "maintains that high satisfaction in old age is usually present in those individuals who accept the inevitability of reduction in social and personal interactions"—in those who disengage from such activities (Busse & Blazer, 1980c). The *activity theory,* on the other hand, holds that "the maintainance of activity is important to most individuals as a basis for obtaining and maintaining satisfaction, self-esteem, and health" (Busse & Blazer, 1980).

On the relevance of activity to successful aspects of aging, several interesting observations have been reported more recently. "Contrary to popular contention, cognitive, not motor, activities showed the highest relationship to general health and longevity" (Burrus-Bammel & Bammel, 1985, p. 858). Moreover, "a significant positive relationship was also found between cognitive recreation activities and intellectual performance," while "activities of a cognitive, affective, and sensory-motor nature separately and combined, showed significant relationships to mental health" (Burrus-Bammel & Bammel, 1985, p. 858). These observations are consistent with findings from the Duke Longitudinal Study on Aging, where Palmore presented data showing that the strongest predictor of successful aging—along an activity/disengagement axis—among both men and women was "secondary-group activity"; major secondary-group activities included "time filled with many groups, much reading, always on the go or occupied with reading, etc." (Palmore, 1979, p. 428).

Considering the above research and my own study of mentally healthy older adults, one cannot help but be impressed with the role of *cognitive* activities apart from *physical* ones in affecting outlook, coping, and life satisfaction in later life. Whereas much conventional wisdom advises us to "keep active" as we age, what is enormously underappreciated is the predominant position of *activities of the mind* in helping people age well. Of course, cognitive and physical activities combined are that much better.

The development of a social portfolio of interests, activities, and interpersonal relationships mentioned before is relevant here. The activities planning grid illustrated in Figure 3.1 offers one approach to planning such a portfolio. The grid is structured along two axes—one that

	COGNITIVE ACTIVITIES	PHYSICAL ACTIVITIES
INDIVIDUAL ACTIVITIES	Reading Writing autobiography	Walking Swimming
GROUP ACTIVITIES	Photo club Elder hostel	Tennis Dancing

Figure 3.1 Activities planning grid.

balances cognitive and physical activities, the other balancing individual
and group efforts. Thus those in later life, who, because of physical
changes are less likely to be able to participate in as many physically
demanding activities, will be well prepared with a solid cognitive
backup. Similarly, those older individuals with less physical mobility and
thinned social networks will have a well grounded backup of individual
activities to rely on in the face of fewer group interchanges. The planning
itself of the grid could be an individual as well as a family endeavor.
Filling in the grid leaves one with a set of four categories of activities—
individual cognitive, group cognitive, individual physical, and *group
physical* activities. The examples provided for each category illustrate
only a few of numerous activities that could be developed. The grid can
also be adapted to accommodate disability as well as health; for example,
if one had rheumatoid arthritis severe enough to interfere with writing,
an autobiography could still be accomplished by an oral taping instead.

SEX AND AGING

How much is sex on the minds and in the actions of older adults? In so
many aspects of aging, images cling to a negative mythology about an
inevitability of decline and eventual disappearance of key capacities. Sex
among the elderly has long been regarded like a vanishing species. This,
too, is untrue. Love and libido and their translation into action among the
aging are the rule rather than the exception.

Interestingly, the Old Testament offers a positive myth to keep hope if
not expectation alive here. In Genesis, Abraham and Sarah find themselves childless in their later years. Abraham, in his 70s, and Sarah, not
quite as old, hear from God that they are going to have a child. Fearful and
full of doubt Sarah gives her husband Abraham her maidservant, Hagar, so
that Hagar might bear a child for them; a child is born and named Ishmael.

Again God promises Abraham and Sarah a son. Sarah musters her courage and at age 90 (Abraham is 100) she gives birth to a son, Isaac.

As with so many other areas in aging, sexuality knows no endpoint in the life cycle, though here, too, changes cannot be denied. The issue, however, is once again that capacity for continuing fulfillment for many, and new opportunities for others, must not be overlooked just because of chronological age. As Comfort (1980) has pointed out, "there are many couples in their 70s who have for the first time achieved communication and fulfillment which had previously been denied them."

Cohort effects, nevertheless, should be kept in mind when analyzing data on sexual interest and activity of the elderly. Today's older adults, for example, did not grow up during the "sexual revolution" of the 1960s and 1970s. Davidson (1985) reminds one of this backdrop in reviewing data on the relatively high proportion of men and women over 80 who remain sexually active. He describes one study of approximately 80 men and 80 women over the age of 80, where sexual intercourse "at least several times a year" was described by 52% of the men and 27% of the women. He notes further that "these individuals spent their formative years in a period of history noted for its prudity and general antagonism to nonprocreative sex."

Comfort reminds us further about the additional variables of "opportunity" (as opposed to ability) affecting sexual encounter as well as the impact of illness (as opposed to aging per se) in interfering with sexual performance. "Asexuality in later life is now known to reflect, as a rule, not the loss of capacity but absence of opportunity, particularly in older women, whose sexual capacity changes little with time, but whose social opportunities are culturally and demographically curtailed with those of older men . . . With women, there is no evidence that the capacity for orgasm declines at any age, and women are known to have become orgasmic for the first time at ages in excess of 80" (Comfort, 1980). As for men, Comfort emphasizes that "it can be said with confidence that impotency is never a consequence of chronological age alone. Its frequency with age is due to a variety of causes"; disease or drug side effects are often implicated here, though the most frequent factors are psychological in nature and often lend themselves to counseling interventions (Butler, 1975; Masters & Johnson, 1981). In other words, rather than looking at life's calendar as an explanation of significant change in sexual interest and activity, psychosocial and biomedical factors should be considered first. There are an increasing number of clinics and clinicians who have the sensitivity and understanding required to evaluate sexual concerns or problems of older adults, and a growing number of therapeutic approaches at hand.

Comfort, reflecting a concern about cohort factors similar to those expressed by Davidson, stresses the need for longitudinal studies where the same individuals can be followed over time. The relevance of this approach is again dramatically illustrated with one group of older adults followed over a five-year period in which 16% reported a falling-off of sexual activity, while 14% reported an *increase* (Comfort, 1980).

The Duke Longitudinal Study of Aging reported that "although older people experienced a decline in sexual activity and strength of sexual drive, these data show that, given the conditions of reasonably good health and partners who are also physically healthy, elderly persons continue to be sexually active into their seventh, eighth, and ninth decades" (Newman & Nichols, 1970). The fact that there were older individuals who experienced increased sexual interest and activity in later life was also found (Verwoerdt, Pfeiffer, & Wang, 1970). The Duke data along with other longitudinal and cross-sectional findings about sexuality in later life have also been looked at from a longitudinal state of mind perspective. Comfort has looked at such data as not reflecting the effect of age as much as an attitudinal and life pattern response, where those who have always been more interested and active in sex are more likely to maintain sexual interest and activity in later life than those who have always been less oriented in this direction. "What we are seeing is not so much an 'age change' as the experience of a mixture of high- and low-activity individuals, in whom those whose sexual 'set' is low for physical or attitudinal reasons drop out early, often with recourse to age as an excuse" (Comfort, 1980).

Butler addresses the potential changes in sexual behavior and opportunity in later life that can come with changes in cultural orientation. The risk has become high of a woman losing her spouse in later life, for two reasons: (1) women have a greater average life expectancy than men, and (2) men tend to be older than their wives—compounding the differential life expectancy problem. This is, of course, a major reason why older women as a whole experience a reduction of opportunity for sexual encounter—less opportunity due to loss of spouse and less availability of older men in general. There is some evidence, though, that age patterns around marriage are showing less cultural rigidity, with some reversal from the classic older husband/younger wife pattern. "For instance, of 450,000 marriages in West Germany in 1973, about 70,000 occurred between an older wife and a younger husband. In Britain that pattern is said to have increased some tenfold in recent years; in Sweden, twelvefold" (Butler, 1975).

From my own study of mentally healthy older persons, variation seems to be the name of the game—a common finding in so many facets of life, particularly in the later years. For those without a spouse, the lack of an easily accessible sexual partner not only affects the opportunity for sexual activity, but it also appears to have an effect on sexual interest. Psychological mechanisms of defense serve to protect us against frustration and disappointment, among which can be the perceived loss of sexual opportunity. Consciously or unconsciously, placing sexual interest on a back burner under such circumstances can be an understandable and adaptive self-protective response on the part of an older person. Waning sexual interest on the part of many older people can then be looked at as an *effect* rather than the cause of diminished sexual activity. While some adapt in this manner, others do not—the latter becoming more motivated for alternatives (e.g., new sexual relationships) or in need of professional consultation. Of course, the frequency of sexual intercourse is certainly not the only way to measure a sense of sexual well being at any point along the life cycle. Expressions of love, affection, sensuality, and sexuality can all mix differently in different individuals and still add up to a sense of emotional fulfillment. Overlooked is the number of people for whom this mix best fits together in their later years.

Still, state of mind factors as they affect love and libido in later life can be complex and intense. The following case example illustrates this situation.

An 83-year-old man, Mr. Obrey, was referred for psychiatric consultation by an activities coordinator at a recreational facility due to concerns about the man's intermittently depressed moods, troubled preoccupation, and a slow but continuing loss of weight. Mr. Obrey appreciated the referral and accepted the appointment that had been arranged.

He described that his wife had died two and a half years earlier, after they had been happily married for 53 years. After a year and a half had passed since his wife's death, he sold his house and moved into a "senior citizen's apartment building" at the suggestion of his son and daughter who thought this would lessen his burdens and improve his social opportunities. Mr. Obrey explained that he frequently thought about his wife, and that for the first 18 months after her death he was very distracted by memories of their life together; they were good memories, but sadness over losing her weighed heavily on him. His appetite had been poor and he had lost weight, but this was improving—until recently. He was otherwise in very good general health with only a mild cardiac arrhythmia, well controlled with medication. Discussion focused further on the more recent resumption of weight loss.

Not long after Mr. Obrey had moved into his new apartment, a neighbor down the hall knocked on his door one day with a casserole of lasagna, just out of the oven. She seemed very pleasant, and Mr. Obrey invited her in as they introduced themselves. They struck up a friendship which over time evolved into romantic feelings. Mr. Obrey began to experience the reawakening of sexual feelings, but was confronted with a sense of guilt about being unfaithful to his wife. It was at this point that his weight loss resumed. His children had met his new friend, took a liking to her, and encouraged their father to further develop the relationship—kidding him encouragingly about his new romantic opportunities. Two months before he came for professional help he did attempt to make love to her, but experienced problems maintaining an erection. He explained that she was very understanding and encouraging. They tried several times after that, with some improvement on his part, but the return of the more distracting thoughts about his wife and the weight loss were starting to bother him even more.

In evaluating Mr. Obrey a thorough general medical examination was also arranged. There appeared to be no physical explanation for his impotency, nor did he seem to be experiencing any side effects from his medication. The most likely reason for his sexual difficulties seemed to be psychogenic. Weekly psychotherapy sessions were scheduled over the next two months. During that period he was able to verbalize the deep ambivalence he had about a new intimate relationship and was able to recognize that thoughts about his wife were particularly prominent when he was about to make love to his new friend. Intellectually he realized that his family and friends were very supportive of his new relationship and that some had even intimated that he was marriage material; he needed more time though to have his emotions catch up. Mr. Obrey did well in therapy, reporting after a month that he was starting to gain weight and even being able to joke that this would be good in building up strength for his love life. By the end of the second month he had taken major steps in coming to terms with his new situation, and reflected at times that his wife would probably be pleased for him. At the same time he was beginning to experience improved sexual performance. Psychotherapy continued over the next several months, but with gradually diminishing frequency.

After about four months had gone by Mr. Obrey came in one day with a very different concern. With some hesitation and stammering he asked, "how often" would be OK, given both his age and his heart condition; by the time he finished therapy after about a year, he figured the "exercise" would be good for both.

This case illustrates three important ways in which one's frame of mind can affect sexual experience and well-being in later life. The confusion, anxiety, and guilt that can accompany the development of a new intimate relationship after the death of one's spouse is vividly shown (with men, sexual problems in this context have been referred to as "Widower's Syndrome" (Masters & Johnson, 1981)). The negative effect on the sexual activity of the elderly from fear of medical complications, particularly about heart strain, is also apparent. It is very important for older individuals to specifically ask their doctors for clarity about any limitations their illnesses or treatments might have on their sexuality. It is equally important for clinicians to anticipate these concerns and without having to be asked, clarify them. Fears of medical risks are typically greatly exaggerated, and usually unfounded. Also illustrated with Mr. Obrey is the recurring theme of disorder (in this case depression), not aging, causing the fundamental problem. The corollary to this theme is also demonstrated—reversibility.

As a closing thought in reviewing the studies to date of sexual interest and activity among the elderly, it should be interesting to see how sexuality in later life unfolds for those who reached sexual maturity during and since the 1960s. As Comfort (1980) put it, "a generation with high sexual expectations, exposed to modern attitudes and counseling and devoid of the expectations of decrepitude, will probably score a great deal higher."

4

Interrelationships Between the Aging Brain and the Aging Body

Given the high prevalence of somatic illness in later life, one is more likely to find a greater interplay of mental and physical disorders in the elderly as compared to other age groups; that is, mental illness is less likely to occur in isolation in older adults than in younger ones. Accordingly, research on older patients is likely to present us with a wealth of new information on the nature of interactions between psychological and somatic factors as they affect illness and well being. Such studies can expand the new frontier of scientific interest around the interface of health and behavior, adding new pieces to this puzzle. Through a focus on aging, we can gain further clues about the influence of the brain on the body, of one's mind on one's matter.

Here we confront one of the most important "sleepers" on the public health front—the impact of psychological state and mental status on the course of overall health and physical illness in later life, the influence of psyche on soma with aging. Many older persons living in the community have the same degree of physical disability as those residing in nursing homes. What makes the difference? Often it is the impact of concomitant psychosocial problems or psychiatric disorder that becomes the straw that breaks the individual's capacity to maintain a more independent level of functioning. The relevance to rehabilitation cannot be overstated (Brody & Ruff, 1986; Williams, 1984). Consider the challenge of a frail older person attempting to manage several medications prescribed for various physical ailments; add a deep depression or psychosis to this and the individual's ability to maintain clarity or organization of thought in managing these drugs may become impaired, with potentially serious consequences to overall health status.

The following case example illustrates in more detail the dynamic interplay that can occur between mental and physical health factors in later life, as well as the possible effect on one's clinical if not life course. The profound influence that emotional factors can have on the progression of physical illness in the elderly becomes apparent; as a corollary, the potentially significant impact of psychiatric intervention on improving the level of an older person's physical and cognitive functioning is also demonstrated.

Case Example: A 91-year-old woman, Ms. Milton, was evaluated in a skilled nursing unit where she had been placed because of severe confusion and weakness that led to falling. The family requested the evaluation to determine whether she had Alzheimer's disease and/or would require nursing home residence from that point on. A detailed history and comprehensive physical and mental evaluations revealed a history of cardiac arrhythmia dating back several years and depression over the past several months. The depression had altered the woman's perception of her situation, making her resentful of the gradually increasing degree with which she was becoming dependent on others for various forms of assistance. It appeared that this resentment extended to her medication, where Ms. Milton had grown more and more annoyed about the number and frequency of medications she had to take. In her depressed state she rebelled against several perceived areas of external controls on her, and, unfortunately, included her antiarrhythmic medicine in the process. When she failed to properly use the heart drug, Ms. Milton's arrhythmia became more pronounced, which resulted in altered blood flow and oxygenation of the brain. This in turn contributed to the confusion she was experiencing and to the difficulty with falls.

When I evaluated the patient in the skilled nursing unit, my impression was that her clinical state had already begun to improve, a factor of her cardiac medications being properly administered. As we talked, I asked her if she had ever met with a psychiatrist before. Her confusion had lifted sufficiently to allow a cryptic response, not clear as to whether it represented a compliment or a critique: "Not of your calibre," she said, with a slight grin. She then explained that while she had conversed with psychiatrists socially, this was her first clinical visit, which she thought was a good thing given her immediate condition.

During the next few weeks, both the confusion and the tendency to fall progressively diminished. Ms. Milton seemed relieved to be able to acknowledge and talk about her depression. She responded very well to supportive psychotherapy, and with the further resolution of her mental state of confusion, returned to her apartment after a two-month stay in the nursing home. Psychiatric treatment continued on an outpatient basis. Two years later, at age 93, her health status was still stable, and in two areas had further improved. With the depression, she had lost her motivation to attend appropriately to the hearing and vision problems she was experiencing. As her mood disorder lifted, she became motivated to acquire a hearing aid and a new pair of glasses, and felt in better contact with her environment.

One of her greatest satisfactions with the progress she experienced was her renewed ability to read and recite from memory some of her favorite Shakespearean sonnets that she had taught during her 40 year career as an English teacher. I asked her one day if she could read me her favorite. Not requiring the book she recited from memory the full fourteen-line sonnet in perfect iambic pentameter:

> That time of year thou mayst in me behold,
> When yellow leaves, or none, or few do hang
> Upon those boughs which shake against the cold,
> Bare ruined choirs, where late the sweet birds sang.
> In me thou seest the twilight of such day,
> As after sunset fadeth in the west,
> Which by and by black night doth take away,
> Death's second self that seals up all in rest.
> In one thou seest the glowing of such fire,
> That on the ashes of his youth doth lie,
> As the death-bed, whereon it must expire,
> Consumed with that which it was nourished by.
> This thou perceiv'st which makes thy love more strong.
> To love that well, which thou must leave ere long.
>   SHAKESPEARE, *Sonnet 73*

Ms. Milton herself commented on the enormous impact her state of mind had on her overall health.

PARADIGMS FOR EXAMINING CONNECTIONS BETWEEN PHYSICAL AND MENTAL HEALTH IN THE ELDERLY

Clinical concerns and research questions pertaining to connections between mental and physical health in the elderly can be framed in a number of ways. Four useful paradigms are (Cohen, 1985b):

1. The impact of severe psychological stress leading to physical health consequences.

    then, its converse,

2. The effect of physical disorder that leads to psychiatric disturbance.

    then, the two together,

3. The effect of coexisting mental and physical disorders on the clinical course of each other.

   and a variation on the former,

4. The influence of psychosocial factors on the clinical course of physical health problems.

These four paradigms will now be elaborated in more detail. In each model, major public health problems of the elderly will provide the illustrations.

1. The impact of severe psychological stress leading to physical health consequences

Example: Depression → Loss of appetite, Anemia, Dehydration

   In addition to the dysphoric mood and discouraged thoughts that typically accompany depression, there may be loss of appetite (anorexia) and less energy to carry out everyday tasks (such as meal preparation). When severe, anorexia in frail older persons can rather quickly lead to altered metabolism, with added jeopardy to physical health status. Dehydration with associated weakness could occur; an anemia could result, adding to the loss of energy caused by the mood disorder; an electrolyte imbalance could be caused, leading to an insidious onset of confusion that could mimic Alzheimer's disease.

2. The effect of physical disorder that leads to psychiatric disturbance

Example: Hearing loss → Onset of delusions

   Approximately one in four elderly individuals has a significant hearing problem (Ruben, 1978). As we will see in Chapter 5, a sensory deprivation phenomenon may be inducing psychotic symptoms in certain vulnerable individuals; loss of hearing has also been described as a possible risk factor in *paraphrenia* (late onset schizophrenia). Research could contribute to a better understanding of which hearing impaired elderly are at risk for developing delusional ideation in later life.

3. The effect of coexisting mental and physical disorders on the clinical course of each other

Example: Congestive heart failure + Depression → Further cardiac decline

Cardiac disease and depression are two of the most common health problems of the elderly. A covert depression (described fully in Chapter 5) could be bringing about indirect suicidal behavior, acted out by the patient through failure to follow a proper schedule of medication. Though further deterioration in overall cardiac capacity might comprise the predominant clinical picture, the major change factor would be the depression.

4. **The influence of psychosocial factors on the clinical course of physical health problems**

Example: An elderly diabetic with an infected foot, living in isolation → Increased risk of developing complications leading to amputation

The absence of adequate social supports can complicate the management of major and chronic physical illnesses. Practically everyone can benefit from having caring others who are supportive and keep the pressure up to maintain diligence in following required medical regimens. That one in seven older men and one in three older women in the U.S. lives alone highlights the need to pay extra attention to the social situation of patients with medical problems in later life. This certainly applies to older diabetics for whom adequate rigor in monitoring the diabetes enhances the ability to control it and to prevent complications such as neglected foot infections which can lead to gangrene and amputation.

There are, of course, many other ways in which research and clinical considerations can focus on the interaction of mental and physical stresses as they affect overall health in later life (Habot & Libow, 1980). Meanwhile, the above paradigms reflect the diversity and potential magnitude of public health problems brought about by such an interplay. Another construct for examining these connections is to take a systems of the body approach—to explore relationships between psychological and physiological phenomena, as within the cardiovascular system of the body, the gastrointestinal system, the endocrine system, the respiratory system, and so forth, in older patients. An example follows with the gastrointestinal system; this example also illustrates a not uncommon diagnostic dilemma in the elderly—the challenge of determining whether the basis for a clinical problem is mental or physical.

WHICH IS IT—MENTAL OR PHYSICAL?

In diagnosing the older patient it is not just a matter of recognizing certain clinical changes as representing the manifestations of illness, but recognizing the right changes—the correct illness. The correct diagnosis can be especially challenging when it comes to differentiating psychological causes from physical ones. Consider gastrointestinal (GI) complaints. This is an interesting example, because it illustrates very well the difficulty confronting many clinicians when examining elderly patients. GI or abdominal complaints comprise an area where one witnesses competing stereotypes at work to explain clinically what is causing the patient's problems. In one camp, the stereotype holds that at the bottom of most GI complaints in the elderly lies a psychogenic origin—a hypochondriachal explanation. The opposite camp believes that if you look hard enough a physical basis will be found to explain most GI symptoms in older patients. Which is correct?

The answer can be found in research. In an attempt to resolve these discrepant views an important study was conducted on 300 patients over age 65 who presented with GI complaints at the outpatient department of a medical center; they were studied comprehensively for at least a year following their initial visit (Sklar, 1978). The various diagnoses that were made and the percentage of patients possessing each diagnosis are listed in the findings that follow:

10% had gastrointestinal malignancy
 8% had bladder disease
 6% had duodenal ulcer
 3% had gastric ulcer
 3% had diverticulosis of the colon
14% had a wide variety of problems with an organic (physical) basis
56% had gastrointestinal distress associated with psychogenic factors, with no anatomical changes to account for them. This category included problems like irritable colon, spastic colitis, gastritis, heart burn, nausea, diarrhea, constipation, and other psychophysiologic problems

In short, the findings reveal that both psychogenic (56%) and physical factors (44%) play major roles in different patients with GI problems, in a ratio of almost 50:50. The clinical significance of these results is that the responsibility of the practitioner—primary care physician or psychiatrist—is equally great to carry out comprehensive general medical and psychiatric workups in evaluating GI complaints in these patients. Patients with GI symptoms often have very different diagnoses.

By pursuing a systems of the body approach, a practical framework is provided not only for clarifying clinical relationships but also for raising new research questions. A further example concerning the respiratory system follows which focuses on raising questions for research. Since geriatrics is still a young field, new hypotheses are in great demand, particularly to explain how psyche interacts with soma in later life. Indeed, much of current thinking about mind/body relationships is of a theoretical nature.

Theoretical Connections Between Depression and Certain Cases of Pneumonia in Older Adults

The fifth leading cause of death in the elderly is pulmonary disease, and within this broad category pneumonia is a major killer. While pneumonia can be caused by any of a number of infectious agents, the pathway to this illness might start before the offending pathogen invades the lungs. Infection involves more than exposure to dangerous bacteria or viruses; it also involves vulnerability. To the extent that an older person develops less physiologic resistance, vulnerability to illness rises. Moreover, psychological factors as well as physical ones can play a part in influencing vulnerability. This can be applied to the pulmonary system and to pneumonia. Consider the following potential pathway to pneumonia.

Depression, itself a major disorder in the elderly, is associated with increased alcohol intake (Simon, 1980). Drinking can represent an effort to dilute sorrow. But alcohol excess in the elderly can have potentially serious consequences in altering normal bodily mechanisms of defense against infection along the respiratory tract (Freeman, 1978). Four basic mechanisms of defense may be challenged:

1. The cough reflex may become impaired by alcohol, thereby reducing the elimination of infected material along the upper respiratory tract (nasopharynx) (Berkowitz, Reichel, & Shim, 1973).
2. Dehydrating properties of alcohol can lead to a drying up of mucus along the respiratory tract, reduced amounts of mucus being less effective in capturing inhaled pathogens for removal via coughing or swallowing.
3. Along the respiratory tract can be found *macrophages,* specialized cells which kill bacteria. How these macrophages are affected by aging is not clear, but alcohol excess has been shown to have a toxic effect on macrophages, rendering them no longer bactericidal (Freeman, 1978).
4. *Cilia* are microscopic finger-like projections lining the respiratory tract. Moving together like a wave, cilia facilitate the upward and outward expulsion of pathogens. There is some suspicion that alcohol excess retards ciliary movement.

Thus, by interfering with the cough reflex, mucus level, macrophage activity, and ciliary movement, alcohol excess can place the older person at greater vulnerability for respiratory tract infections. Furthermore, alcohol acts like a drug for the elderly in that it takes a lesser amount to reach toxic levels than in earlier adulthood; the decrease in body water which accompanies aging results in higher blood levels of alcohol. Aging, therefore, compounds the effect of alcohol on the normal mechanisms of defense along the respiratory tract.

Awareness of this possible scenario—of depression leading to alcohol excess, which in turn raises the risk of respiratory tract infection—has relevance to both clinical practice and prevention. The physician's perspective should be expanded when treating older patients with recurrent colds, episodes of bronchitis, or bouts of pneumonia. With some of these patients, an underlying depression or alcohol abuse may be the catalyst of illness. The ramifications for proper diagnosis, treatment, and prevention of future occurrences are apparent. The point about prevention is important. In this case we can see how in dealing with psychological and behavioral problems one could possibly lower the risk for physical disorder; this corresponds to the first paradigm above. By working on the aging psyche, we might help the aging soma.

This example offers a variation on the "is it mental or physical" question. It addresses the sequence of psychological and somatic factors and their effect on clinical course.

MENTAL AND PHYSICAL FACTORS ACTING IN COMBINATION IN THE ELDERLY

In addition to the special knowledge base that applies to geriatrics, an aspect that typically distinguishes older patients in general from younger ones is their greater likelihood to be experiencing more than one illness and to be receiving more than one treatment at the same time. Moreover, this mix of illnesses commonly combines mental and physical problems. Hence, an older patient may be suffering from heart disease and depression, while being treated with antihypertensive and antidepressant medications. Elderly patients are a rich resource in helping us to better understand the interaction of different illnesses and the interaction of different treatments (e.g., drug–drug interactions). They may be our best reminder of the need to treat the *whole* person.

Case Example: Mrs. LaRue, an 82-year-old widow living by herself in an efficiency apartment, was referred for evaluation because of memory changes described as "so severe that she could not even recall the death of a daughter who had died two months earlier." The two had been extremely close, with the daughter visiting her mother almost every other day over a period of many months. The patient was also characterized as being constantly fatigued and not wanting to eat. Her son-in-law, who helped to arrange the consultation, was worried that Mrs. LaRue was becoming "senile," and he was concerned that nursing home placement might become necessary. From this history one might wonder whether Mrs. LaRue was suffering an acute major depressive reaction, given the loss of a very close daughter on whom she had grown quite dependent, and given the symptoms of fatigue and anorexia that frequently accompany severe depressions. The possibility of pseudodementia became an important consideration.

I visited Mrs. LaRue in her apartment. In response to a knock on the door, a faint voice from inside said to come in, that the door was not locked. Upon entering, I found Mrs. LaRue lying on her couch, motioning me to come over to her. My eyes quickly scanned her apartment. The place appeared in a slight disarray, and an empty wine bottle was observed under a corner table beside the couch. Pulling up a chair, I sat down beside the patient. She looked lethargic, with dry skin, and as she spoke she seemed dispirited.

As our discussion proceeded I indicated my understanding that her daughter had recently died and how it must have been a very painful loss for her, and I asked what had led to her daughter's death. She did not respond to the question, appearing as if she could not comprehend it, and went on to another topic. One could easily be suspicious of cognitive impairment, of a dementing process. Noticing on a nearby bureau a photograph that appeared to be a family portrait, I brought it over to the patient to discuss it with her. Curiously, she was able to provide a reasonable family history for each person in the picture except one who she could not recall—the recently deceased daughter. Half an hour later, as I was getting up to leave, Mrs. LaRue spontaneously broke into tears and began to tell me about her daughter, as if I had just asked the question.

Mrs. LaRue was able to convey that her daughter had suffered from a cardiac condition that led to hospitalization for heart surgery. Unexpectedly, the daughter died from complications following the operation. At that point a case could have been made for a psychogenic basis for the patient's symptoms. She looked and sounded depressed, manifesting symptoms of loss of energy and appetite consistent with a diagnosis of depression. In addition, she had suffered a major loss that could have precipitated a major mood disorder.

Thinking about her difficulty in responding to questions about her daughter's death and the dramatic *isolated* lack of recognition with the family portrait, a psychodynamic explanation for her seeming cognitive impairment could be proposed: Because the patient had become extremely dependent on her daughter, Mrs. LaRue experienced her daughter's death not only as a tragic loss but unconsciously as a form of abandonment as well. She was left then with mixed feelings of both grief and anger—angry over being abandoned. But how could she be angry at this daughter whom she had so loved and who had been so devoted to her? Unable to deal with this distressing ambivalence, such disturbingly mixed feelings, Mrs. LaRue psychologically repressed thoughts of her daughter's death. The price she paid for bottling up these painful feelings was clinical depression, and by blocking out emotionally charged memories this depression mimicked dementia. This was my initial synthesis.

But there was additional information to be gleaned. One could see that the patient was clearly dehydrated, that she had been eating very poorly, while suspicion of drinking was raised by the empty and casually discarded wine bottle. That geriatric patients commonly have more than one clinical problem operating at the same time also had to be considered. The next step, therefore, was a comprehensive general medical workup. The results indicated that the patient had marked dehydration, an iron deficiency anemia, and a duodenal ulcer.

Upon reconsideration, six clinical problems were identified—all treatable. Mrs. LaRue was clearly (1) depressed; (2) it appeared that alcohol abuse associated with the depression was also playing a part; (3) the patient was dehydrated, (4) anemic, and (5) had an ulcer, possibly aggravated by the stress associated with the daughter's death; (6) she was also in a social crisis, needing in-home assistance to compensate for the loss of help she had been receiving from her daughter. In re-examining her major symptoms of confusion, fatigue, and appetite disturbance, the explanation for each could be expanded. The confusion was probably a factor of both the depression and the dehydration, influenced, too, by the alcohol; the fatigue could be explained by the depression in combination with the anemia and dehydration; the appetite disturbance was likely caused by the depression and drinking, compounded by the ulcer.

A problem-oriented treatment plan based on the six clinical problems was instituted. Brief hospitalization resulted in rapid rehydration. Homemaker assistance was arranged to assure adequate hydration, nutritional intake, and assistance with household chores. Medications were prescribed to treat the ulcer and anemia. Psychotherapy was instituted, helping the patient work through her depression and to overcome the drinking problem.

This case is a good illustration of the multifactorial basis for much illness in the elderly. It is a good reminder to avoid the pitfalls of a narrow either/or approach in seeking a single cause to explain clinical symptoms in the geriatric patient. The positive treatment opportunities that accompany awareness of mind/body interactions with aging are also apparent.

MENTAL SYMPTOMS SIGNALING PHYSICAL ILLNESS IN THE ELDERLY

What information does the state of the aging mind give us about the state of the aging body? The relationship of a sound mind in later life to increased longevity has long been noted; in particular, sustained intellectual functioning with aging has been well correlated with enhanced survival (Granick, 1971; Jarvik & Falek, 1963). Conversely, significant change in intellectual performance typically signals underlying illness, Alzheimer's disease being one of the most serious examples. Other mental changes in later life may also be an indication of underlying disorder—often of a physical nature. Depression, for example, may signal cancer (Rodin & Voshart, 1986).

Carcinoma of the pancreas is one of the classic examples where depression may be the first symptom of a covert cancer (Jarvik & Perl, 1981). While in some cases, psychiatric manifestations of cancer may be the result of metastasis of the tumor to the brain, different explanations have been postulated in other cases (Whitlock & Siskind, 1979).

Scientific Speculation Leading to New Frontiers of Research

One of the most intriguing among the other explanations for depression, still speculative in nature, requires knowledge of the biogenic amine theory of depression (discussed in the next chapter). In simple terms, the *biogenic amine hypothesis* holds that a depletion of certain neurotransmitters results in a depressed mood; norepinephrine and serotonin are the neurotransmitters most implicated in studies to date. Since these neurotransmitters function by interacting with receptor sites in the brain, if those receptor sites were blocked, the result would be similar to the neurotransmitter being depleted.

Based on some preliminary data from animal studies, it has been hypothesized that the body develops antibodies against early developing cancer cells. However, these data also suggest that some of these antibodies may additionally interact with the receptor sites in the brain that receive the neurotransmitter serotonin (Brown & Paraskevas, 1982). As a consequence, the suspected cross-reactivity of these antibodies could be blocking the access of serotonin to its receptor sites. This in turn would simulate a state of serotonin depletion in the brain, resulting in depression. Unlike the case of a brain metastasis, though, this depression could be occurring much earlier in the course of the cancer, thereby increasing the chance of earlier recognition and treatment of the hidden malignancy. That cancer is the second leading cause of death in the elderly makes this line of investigation not only interesting but highly relevant in potentially identifying more timely therapeutic options. Such research is part of one of the most exciting new frontiers in psychiatry— the relationship of mental phenomena to the body's immune system. At the least, inquiry of this nature can broaden the reach of our questions.

While the theory just presented focuses on the possibility of immune changes affecting mental functioning, the opposite is also being studied, namely, the negative impact of mental disorder on immunologic functioning. Thus there have been studies that have attempted to determine if depression has any causal relationship to cancer. The results have been conflicting, with some researchers finding no increase in malignancies among those with mood disorders (Evans, Baldwin, & Gath, 1974; Niemi & Jaaskelainen, 1978), while other investigators have reported that a connection may exist (Whitlock & Siskind, 1979; Shekelle, Raynor, Ostfeld, et al., 1981). Considerably more research needs to be done in this area, on the relation of depression and stress in general to cancer and immunologic functioning (Shavit, Terman, Martin, et al., 1985).

A Relationship Between Bereavement and Mortality in Later Life

To the extent that linkages between mental and physical health can be further recognized and their mechanisms better understood, new opportunities for preventive clinical interventions can be identified. One such area that has received considerable attention is conjugal bereavement surrounding the death of a spouse. Such loss is regarded as among the most potentially stressful of commonly occurring life events, and has been associated with increased medical illness and mortality in the surviving spouse (Jacobs & Ostfeld, 1977). Because of the strong relationship here between psychological stress and increased risk to overall health, particular attention has been focused on this group of at-risk individuals in studying possible connections between depression and immunologic dysfunction (Stein, Keller, & Schleifer, 1985). Again, it is the elderly who are the main subjects in this research—the group that has provided one of the best windows to study this phenomenon, to the benefit of all age groups.

Following the finding that the death of one spouse was accompanied by an increased frequency of physical illness and mortality in the other, further research compared the impact on surviving husbands with that of surviving wives (Jacobs & Ostfeld, 1977). Women were found to be most affected for as long as two years after the death of a husband; for men, adverse effects were observed to occur almost exclusively within the first six months after losing a wife.

The explanation for this apparent increased vulnerability to physical disorder and death remains a research question, though theories of brain hormone (neuroendocrinologic) involvement are growing (Besedovsky, Del Rey, & Sorkin, 1985; Calabrese, Kling, & Gold, 1987; Pert, Ruff, Weber, et al., 1985; Stein et al., 1985). When people are startled, their bodies respond to make them more alert; their adrenal glands release the hormone adrenaline (epinephrine) which serves to stimulate the body into a state of heightened alertness, as with pupils dilating and the heart pumping faster. This "stress response" is a classical example of the translation of a psychological stimulus into a physical response by the body. Increasingly, it has been found that such endocrinologic responses throughout the body are under the control of the brain, mediated by the hypothalamus and the pituitary gland of the brain. With the identification of a growing number of neurotransmitters and brain hormones, theories of their potential role in affecting not only other endocrine but immune system functions as well are gaining fuel. These theories have led to new investigations that are looking very closely at the effect of severe stress sustained over a considerable period of time, seeking connections between neuroendocrine responses and immune system changes.

While the findings associated with conjugal bereavement are of enormous relevance to the potential understanding of underlying disease processes and connections between mental and physical health phenomena, they are similarly important for treatment. The identification of fairly well defined time intervals of maximum risk for widows and widowers subsequent to the death of a spouse allows for a more rational plan of intervention. Not only is the potential need for intervention around the loss of a husband or wife apparent, but a sense of *how long* extra social supports or treatment should be considered is also provided, along with an awareness of differences between the needs of men and women. In addition to different durations of maximum risk for physical morbidity associated with losing a spouse, suicidal behavior also varies around this problem when comparing men with women. For women rates of suicide associated with widowhood are lower than for men, peaking at about age 50; for men, rates remain high with advancing age. The relevance to more informed program planning in offering help and in exploring possible prevention strategies is again evident. So, too, is the opportunity for older people themselves to take active steps in seeking consultation to either resolve or prevent prolonged bereavement.

What these findings suggest is that prolonged bereavement following the death of a husband or wife is a signal of increased risk for physical morbidity and mortality in the surviving spouse, and one that merits careful attention. Mental symptoms signaling potential or actual physical problems in the elderly remind us of the close relationship between mind and body with aging, and challenge us to not look past them as if they were incidental phenomena.

Case Example: A couple in their 60s came in to discuss the wife's 86-year-old father, Mr. Green, who was living with them during the energy crisis in the early 1970s. They described Mr. Green as slowly developing more and more disturbed thoughts over the past few months. He complained that when his daughter left for work, people would sneak into the house and tamper with the food in the refrigerator. He was also concerned that his phone conversations were being tapped, and that serious trouble was lurking. These concerns were then used as an excuse by him to confine himself to his daughter's home, to stand guard over it rather than visit with his cronies; Mr. Green's friends were also becoming alarmed about his increasingly bizarre behavior. What his daughter and son-in-law described sounded like the insidious onset of paranoid thoughts, an acute psychosis.

In trying to determine the next steps, further background on Mr. Green was gathered from his family. No prior psychiatric history was described; no traumatic events were associated with the onset of his symptoms; no recent changes in his overall medical condition were evident. There was one thing, though, that was finally detected as being different. The family portrayed Mr. Green as always having been both conscientious and frugal, if not slightly eccentric, even as a younger man. More recently he had become quite concerned about the worsening energy crisis and wanted to do something about it, to make a personal contribution or sacrifice.

One day an idea came to him, which he acted on. At this point, as the family related the history, it became apparent that Mr. Green was hard of hearing and that he wore a hearing aid. His idea was that he could set an example for others on how to save energy in creative ways by conserving on the use of the batteries for his hearing aid. For most of the day, he now kept his hearing aid turned off. Within three months of this change, his new symptoms began to emerge. It appeared that Mr. Green had induced a sensory deprivation state for himself, leading to his delusional ideation.

The patient's internist was contacted, and the case reviewed with him. The internist confirmed that Mr. Green's general medical condition had been rather stable, but did not know about the hearing aid idiosyncrasy. The internist felt comfortable in managing the problem himself, with psychiatric consultation on the treatment plan. He was advised that given the magnitude of the patient's paranoia, a low dose of anti-psychotic medication could be prescribed in helping the delusions to more quickly resolve. Meanwhile, Mr. Green was to be carefully coached to find alternative avenues for energy conservation.

He did agree to restore standard usage of his hearing aid. Within a month Mr. Green's symptoms had greatly abated, and were essentially gone by the eighth week of treatment. His anti-psychotic medication was gradually terminated two months later. A follow-up a year later found no return of delusions, and continuing proper use of the hearing aid. The mental symptoms had served to signal an adverse change in the management of a physical problem, though this important connection had not been initially observed.

TREATING THE AGING MIND TO HELP THE AGING BODY—SAVINGS IN SUFFERING AND IN DOLLARS

Some of the best research to show the impact of psychiatric intervention on the course of physical illness has been carried out on the elderly. In a now classic study by Levitan and Kornfeld (1981), the investigators compared the clinical outcomes of two groups of elderly patients who underwent surgery for fractured femurs. The treatment group of 24 patients aged 65 and older received psychiatric consultation during hospitalization, while the control group of 26 patients in the same age group did not receive any psychiatric intervention. The groups were alike in terms of reason for admission (a broken thighbone), age, surgical intervention, hospital setting, and overall medical care—except that one group received psychiatric consultation while the other did not. The group receiving psychiatric attention revealed two major outcome differences from the control group. The treatment group had (1) a substantially shorter length of stay in the hospital, and (2) a significantly improved clinical outcome.

Length of stay was 12 days or 29% shorter for the treatment group when compared to the controls; there was an average hospital stay of 30 days for the former group of patients versus 42 for the latter. Moreover *twice* as many patients in the treatment group returned home rather than being discharged to a nursing home or other health-related institution. From a cost savings perspective, it was calculated that over the course of a year, services for a liaison psychiatrist providing consultation to such patients would cost approximately $10,000, with gross cost savings from shorter lengths of stay and lower frequency of nursing home placements coming to $193,000. This would result in a net cost savings of $183,000 over the course of a year. These findings portray a dramatic influence of the state of one's mind on the response of one's body—in this case, the *aging* body—in the face of major physical trauma. They are far from unique, as reflected in the following review of more than thirty additional studies.

To gain further insight on the influence of attending to the mind on the course of medical as well as surgical problems, a large number of studies that examined the effects of psychologically oriented intervention on recovery from surgery and heart attacks were reviewed (Mumford, Schlesinger, & Glass, 1982). A significant number of patients in these studies were elderly. Thirty-four controlled studies were described in which surgical or coronary patients who, through interpersonal interchange, were provided either information or emotional support to master their medical crisis did better than patients who received only ordinary care; those patients who received both emotional support and information did the best of all. In addition, 13 studies were reviewed in which hospital days post-surgery or post-heart attack were used as outcome measures; findings showed that, on the average, psychologically oriented interventions reduced hospitalization approximately 2 days below that of the control groups' average of 9.92 days (a 20% reduction in length of hospital stay). We see once more the impact of mental health interventions on the course of physical illness. From a dollars perspective in today's cost-conscious society, the results are similarly noteworthy.

The underlying mechanisms that explain the improvement in the clinical course of physical disorders on applying psychiatric interventions are not always clear and seem to vary. For example, a number of patients hospitalized for the treatment of general medical diseases are found to have coexisting, often unidentified, mental health problems. One study found that a remarkable 24% of 406 elderly men seen for physical health reasons in a primary care setting complained of clinically significant depressive symptoms (Boorson, Barnes, Kukull, et al., 1986). Various investigators have long noted that, regardless of diagnostic category, acutely ill older people with mood disorders require more time to recover from physical health problems than patients not suffering from an affective disturbance (Bergmann & Eastman, 1974).

Again, a patholophysiologic basis that will explain how a mental disorder can aggravate the course of a physical illness is often elusive. In the case of heart disease, the number one killer in the elderly, it has been proposed that stress associated with depression or anxiety may accelerate the atherosclerotic process implicated in various cardiac disorders (Moylan & Flye, 1978). But here, too, how stress might effect such acceleration becomes difficult to specify. It may be that psychoimmunologic processes alluded to above play a part in affecting the pace at which damaged or inflamed tissue recovers.

That a mechanism of action cannot be demonstrated does not negate therapeutic effect when it is real and replicable. Many medications, for example, are effective without the basis for their efficacy being understood; this applies to drugs for physical as well as mental disorders. Nonetheless, exciting developments are occurring in the laboratory that are expanding our views on the nature of different links between mental and physical phenomena—on both the dynamics of illness and the basis for treatments (Reiser, 1984). Certainly the role of neurotransmitters in the genesis of depression is a case in point, where chemical imbalances in the brain result in aberrant behavioral manifestations. This discovery has been translated into the development of effective drugs in the treatment of depression, of pharmacologic agents that act through an alleviation of the neurotransmitter deficits.

Preliminary findings from research on psychoimmunology represent another possible link, pointing to the role of stress affecting the release of brain hormones which directly or indirectly appear to influence the response of immune system cells, thereby increasing vulnerability to physical illness. From studies on chronic anxiety, a search for links at the molecular level has raised the possibility of certain structural changes within brain nerve cells (Kandel, 1983). Since nerve cells communicate with one another through the release of neurotransmitters, anxiety may be associated with the increased release of specific chemical communicators. Chronic anxiety may reflect a structural alteration in the size or number of vesicles on nerve cells that store and release these neurotransmitters. The stimulus affecting vesicle status could come from either internal (e.g., genetic expression) or external (e.g., environmental stress) sources, or a combination of these and other factors.

Moving from the molecular level to what meets the eye, other mind–body relationships emerge. Sometimes it is a disturbance of the mind that interferes with necessary attention to a disturbance of the body in the aging patient.

Case Example: The sister of Ms. Waters (a 67-year-old woman with chronic schizophrenia) contacted me with a sense of urgency. The sister described Ms. Waters as being diabetic and having developed an infected foot that was getting worse. But Ms. Waters was refusing to seek medical attention, saying that God was in touch with her, assuring her that He would watch out for her. Her sister knew, however, that Ms. Waters might eventually lose her foot if the infection was not treated. In the past, Ms. Waters had received psychiatric treatment and neuroleptic (antipsychotic) medication, though neither had been utilized during the previous 10 years. Since Ms. Waters would not go to the clinic, I offered to meet with the patient and her sister in Ms. Water's apartment.

Upon being introduced to Ms. Waters by her sister at the apartment, the patient said there was no need for me to be there, that God was looking out for her. She said that I should go and not take up her time. But while so instructing me, she continued to talk about God in a manner that kept up the conversation between us. She then walked across the room and sat down in a chair, reciting that she had nothing else to say. She did not stop talking, however, and selected a chair that was next to an empty one, as if she positioned herself to have someone sit next to her.

Speculating that this was her *nonverbal* message to me, I walked over to the chair and sat down next to her. I felt that while the conscious thoughts on her mind were expressed as verbal resistance, the unconscious ones were conveyed in the form of accepting *body language*. When Ms. Waters registered no nonverbal discomfort I sensed I was on sound footing, even though she reminded me that she did not need any help. I proceeded to explain to her that her foot was badly infected, that an emergency situation with it could develop. I suggested further that she allow her sister to bring her to the internist in the clinic and have treatment initiated. She resumed her litany about God's help, though without suggesting again that I leave.

After about an hour I did leave, and later arranged to have a private consultation with the sister. I reviewed with her the scenario that had transpired and suggested that the sister try escorting the patient to the internist, tactfully ignoring verbal resistance; I recommended against forcing her if she physically resisted, but rather to try again a few days later if necessary. If the patient did not resist, then it would be important to accompany her during the entire visit, gently removing her stocking from her foot to be examined, and so forth. To the sister's astonishment, the pattern of divergent verbal and nonverbal messages persisted, and the visit to the internist was successfully completed, with treatment initiated. The sister was very relieved and wondered how to proceed from there in helping Ms. Waters.

The sister's initial request had not been out of concern about Ms. Waters' psychotic thoughts, but about her physical health. The whole episode, though, forced the sister to reevaluate the situation and to realize that things had deteriorated in the absence of regular psychiatric follow-up for the patient. What made things especially difficult was that Ms. Waters simply refused to take pills, at least on a regular basis. She needed to be on medication.

The sister, who was widowed, was in the process of retiring and was discussing the pooling of resources with another sister also widowed. The two had been thinking about sharing a place together, and now that the concern about Ms. Waters was much greater, they thought that they might try to get her to live with them as well. That way they could not only better watch out for Ms. Waters, but they could all benefit by dividing the costs of a larger living arrangement among them. Ms. Waters went along with the idea. Further consultation among Ms. Waters' two sisters and myself resulted in a plan where I would see the patient on periodic follow-ups, while attempting to have her take neuroleptics in liquid form; the idea again was that her nonverbal acquiescence might allow her to accept the medication in this less apparent manner.

The plan worked fairly well. Eleven years later, the three were still living together, in reasonable compatibility. Ms. Waters had become physically more frail, though her delusions had slightly diminished in intensity. She continued to say that she did not need to see me, but continued to accept my visits.

While most of my work with Ms. Waters had been in the form of brief follow-ups with medication management, it benefited from a psychodynamic orientation as well, drawing upon knowledge of discrepancies between verbal and nonverbal expressions, between stated and unconscious desires. This orientation was essential to successfully reinstituting and maintaining neuroleptic treatment. It also illustrates the problems of attempting to administer drugs without attending to psychological issues. The case itself illustrates the problems that sometimes occur in attempting to treat physical disorder without attending to concurrent psychological disturbance in the elderly.

SOMATIC TREATMENT AND PSYCHIATRIC DISORDER IN THE ELDERLY

This is a two-way street. Drugs can treat psychiatric disorders. Drugs can cause psychiatric disorders. Indeed, dichotomies pervade attitudes and discussions on drug use—on psychotropic drug use in particular. But medications are like so many other things one confronts in life; they are turned to for their assets, while one is aware of their potential liabilities. Drugs are a major issue with the elderly, since far more medications are used by older adults than by any other age group (Lamy, 1980; Nolan & O'Malley, 1988a; Nolan & O'Malley, 1988b). While comprising around 11% of the total U.S. population, those 65 and older have been estimated to make up to 25% of the expenditures on prescription and nonprescription drugs in this country (Vestal, 1985). After prescriptions for cardiovascular problems and pain, psychotropic medications come next, among older patients (Salzman, 1984a). Psychotropic medications include antidepressants, antianxiety agents, antipsychotics (neuroleptics), hypnotics (sleeping medications), lithium (for manic-depressive disorders), and drugs used with the goal of enhancing memory.

Psychotropic drugs have been referred to as everything from "chemical shackles" to "emotional liberators." They have been branded the former when inappropriately or overprescribed, and they have been acclaimed the latter when effective and relieving of symptoms. The fact is, their impact has been historic. Most dramatic were the changes that followed the introduction, in the early 1950s, of the neuroleptic medication chlorpromazine for the treatment of psychosis. Prior to the use of this drug, two-thirds of schizophrenic patients spent most of their lives confined to state mental hospitals; since then, 95% of schizophrenics have been spending most of their time living in the community (Davis, 1985). The combination of neuroleptic medication and the development of community psychiatry resulted in a two-thirds decrease in the state psychiatric hospital population, from 560,000 patients in 1955 to 184,000 in 1977 (Katz, 1985). The elderly have as much opportunity as other age groups to benefit from this progress. But they are too often denied the opportunity, either out of lack of knowledge about psychotropic drug efficacy in older adults or fear that the drugs will not be safe to use. Certainly many of the case examples presented throughout this book reflect the major help psychotropic drugs can offer elderly patients.

Two points are useful in maintaining a proper perspective on drug use, and are helpful in the education and reassurance of the patient:

1. *The Benefit to Risk Ratio:* Drugs are obviously turned to for certain desired effects. Concerns that arise primarily center on their side effects. Unfortunately, as various pharmacologists point out, "a drug that has no side effect, has no effect." It is a rare drug that does just one thing, that has just one effect. An aspirin, for example, does many things. It can relieve pain, fever, itching, etc; it can also cause undesired effects, such as an upset stomach. In most cases side effects are *possible* effects, not *probable* effects of a properly used drug. If serious side effects were inevitable and uncontrollable, the drug would likely not be on the market. To be on the market, drugs need to be both *effective* and *safe* when properly prescribed and utilized. In addition, their potential *benefits* must outweigh their potential *risks.*

2. *Prescribing Patterns versus Utilization Behavior:* Safe and effective drug use is dependent on two behaviors—that of the doctor and that of the patient. Trouble can occur when either fails to follow the proper course. The physician must be diligent about prescribing the right drug at the right dose, while mindful of how the patient's other drugs or other medical conditions might interact with the new prescription. The patient has a responsibility to carefully comply with the prescribed pattern of drug use, while

being diligent in alerting the physician to any problems or questions that arise. Patient compliance can be an enormous problem. A review of over 50 studies found that between 25 and 50% of all outpatients fail to take medications as prescribed (Vestal, 1985). A careful survey of drug-taking patterns in 178 ambulatory patients aged 60 and older revealed that 59% made one or more medication usage errors, the errors being potentially serious in 26% (Vestal, 1985). This is why it is important that when different health care providers come into contact with patients on medications, drug usage be reviewed with the patient; while the physician prescribes the medication, any member of the health care team might play a vital role in monitoring proper drug use in the elderly. Similarly it is important to involve significant others from the older patient's social support system when compliance problems become of concern.

How the Aging Body Handles Drugs for the Troubled Aging Mind

Though psychotropic medications are handled differently as one's body ages, the same efficacy can still be achieved (Nickens, Crook, & Cohen, 1986). In general, when a psychotropic drug is given to an older patient it will usually (though not always) take longer to work, stay longer in the body, and produce a greater effect than it would in a younger person at the same dosage (Salzman, 1982). Given these changes the physician has been advised to "start low, go slow," to begin with a reduced dosage, and to increase it very gradually if necessary. Following this formula, while paying careful attention to potential drug interactions if the patient has other medications or illnesses, will keep the physician on safe and effective footing.

Knowledge of differences in how the aging body handles psychotropic medications fosters a more rational approach to prescribing and monitoring drug use in the elderly. Moreover, the great need to better understand the dynamics of drug action (pharmacokinetics) in the elderly, given their very high utilization of medications in general, has significantly advanced our understanding of pharmacokinetics as a whole. With aging, there are essentially five major areas of pharmacokinetic change (Hollister, 1981; Salzman, 1984a): (1) *absorption* of the drug into the body, (2) *distribution* of the drug throughout the body, (3) *metabolism* of the drug, (4) *excretion* of the drug from the body, and (5) *central nervous system sensitivity* to the drug at receptor sites in the brain.

Absorption. Most psychotropic drugs taken orally by older adults are absorbed through the stomach and intestinal walls. Though the aging process per se does not significantly alter absorption, many older persons are taking prescribed or over-the-counter medications that can interfere with how efficiently or quickly these drugs are absorbed. Antacids and stomach relaxers stand out, each slowing absorption for a different reason. As a result, more attention needs to be paid as to when the psychotropic medication is ingested, perhaps on an empty stomach or an hour earlier before going to bed in order to allow enough time for a hypnotic prescribed for sleep to be absorbed and go to work.

Distribution.   Once a drug is absorbed, it becomes distributed throughout the body. The ratio of body fat to muscle mass and water then becomes important. With aging, body fat tends to increase, while lean muscle mass and water diminish. Except for lithium, all psychotropic medications are lipid (fat) soluble; lithium is water soluble. The increased proportion of fat in the aging body results in the lipid-soluble psychotropic agents being stored in greater quantities and for longer intervals of time, making the same dosage more likely to build up to toxic levels in the older patient as compared to a younger one. This applies even more to older women, since they have proportionately more body fat than older men. The risk of greater drug buildup can be compensated for by lowering the dosage and/ or frequency of usage; it may then take longer for the therapeutic effect to be achieved with lipid-soluble drugs, but the slower pace will result in greater safety. Because the amount of body water decreases with aging, less water-soluble medication (e.g., lithium) is required for the elderly in comparison to younger adults to achieve comparable therapeutic effects.

Metabolism.   Most psychotropic medications, with the exception of lithium, are metabolized or broken down in the liver. As people age, liver metabolism slows due to the altered activity of liver enzymes. If the rate of drug breakdown is reduced, the agent would again tend to stay available and active longer in the body, leading to an increased risk of buildup and toxicity if the same amount continues to be used in later life. Specific knowledge of differences with aging in the rate at which the liver metabolizes various psychotropic medications can be clinically very important. Consider antianxiety agents. Diazepam and chlordiazepoxide are in general metabolized three times more slowly in the old than the young. Oxazepam and lorazepam, on the other hand, are metabolized at essentially the same relatively fast rates regardless of age. Not surprisingly, the latter two are often preferred by geriatric psychiatrists when drugs are indicated for the treatment of anxiety in the elderly, since the risk of them building up in the body is reduced. However, drugs that are rapidly metabolized often need to be taken more frequently. This could create a problem for patients with memory impairment receiving medication for anxiety; they might experience more difficulty remembering to take their drugs. For these patients, a drug that could be taken just once a day might be preferable. It becomes an issue of balancing the risk of one drug that might build up with that of another that might have to be taken too often to be remembered by an impaired patient. In short, having an understanding of underlying drug dynamics allows for greater individualization with older patients when the rote approach with younger ones may no longer apply.

Excretion. While liver metabolism is the primary mechanism for deactivating lipid-soluble psychotropic agents, the water-soluble lithium is deactivated by being excreted from the body via the kidneys. Since the kidneys function more slowly with aging, it takes longer to excrete lithium in the elderly, once again setting the stage for possible build up if dosage is not adjusted downward.

Central Nervous System Sensitivity. The adequacy of reduced levels of psychotropic medications for the elderly in achieving therapeutic effects may also be explained by increased sensitivity at the drugs' sites of action. Here, too, taking the same amount of the drug as one did in earlier adulthood may increase the risk for side effects in the elderly.

Choice of Psychotropic Drug as a Factor of Physical Health Status

Within each category of psychotropic medication, there are several drugs to choose from (Crook & Cohen, 1981; Salzman, 1984a). But the different choices are typically all similar in efficacy. In other words, among the antidepressants, one drug is as therapeutic as the other in alleviating depression in the elderly. How does one choose? The choice is determined as much by side effect to avoid as desired effect to achieve. While similar in effectiveness, drugs differ in the types of side effects they might cause. The nature of the older person's physical health problems, therefore, will determine which psychotropic medication is safest to use. Hence, the choice of drug may differ, depending on the older patient's overall health picture.

For example, all antipsychotic agents can lower blood pressure as a side effect. If an older schizophrenic also has problems with low blood pressure (hypotension), it might be better to use an antipsychotic drug that is less likely to cause hypotensive episodes. Unfortunately, a drug that is less likely to cause one type of side effect may be more likely to cause another. Thus, it is a matter of trade-offs within the broader benefit-versus-risk framework.

In an effort to help focus the choices for clinicians, different publications have attempted to present tables listing drugs in relation to their degree of association with various major side effects, along with other relevant information. Several of these efforts have been adapted in the drug tables that are included in the Appendix.

Antidepressant and Electroconvulsant Therapy in the Elderly

A number of general considerations apply to the use of antidepressant medication in the elderly. There are issues of efficacy, dosage, side effects, and of course the range of drugs to choose from. Again, the choice is typically based on avoiding specific side effects. Table A.3 in the Appendix is designed to delineate most of the major antidepressants, while indicating the side effects of primary concern associated with each drug in older patients. One class of antidepressants (the monamine oxidase inhibitors) is not included in the table and is discussed separately. In addition, electroconvulsant therapy, another form of somatic treatment for depression, is also addressed individually.

Efficacy. The various antidepressants obtained by prescriptions are all similar in potential efficacy, including the "new generation" antidepressants that came on the market more recently.

Dosage. In conditions requiring the most conservative approaches to medicating, most of the antidepressants can be started at even lower doses than commonly suggested (even lower than those indicated in the Table A.3 of the Appendix). In addition, many can be increased in small increments of 10–25 mg at a time. Sometimes dosages greater than those indicated in Table A.3 may be required.

Side Effects. In general, there are four groups of *potential* side effects of most concern with antidepressants: sedation, hypotension, cardiac disturbances, and anticholinergic effects.

Sedation: This effect can be mitigated by administering as much of the medication as possible at bedtime, where the sedation may even alleviate difficulty falling asleep caused by the depression.

Hypotension (low blood pressure): When it occurs, it is often most marked as the patient rises, resulting in momentary dizziness and a risk of falling. Hence, clinicians advise these patients to gradually get up and stand in place for half a minute or so, holding on to a support, to allow their blood pressure to readjust.

Cardiac toxicity: Heart rate and rhythm disturbances can potentially occur, requiring careful monitoring.

Anticholinergic effects: Memory disturbance is one of the potential problems most closely monitored; when it does occur, it is reversible. Other potential problems include dry mouth, urinary difficulties, constipation, blurred vision, and aggravation of glaucoma.

Other considerations: The new generation antidepressants increase one's choices, but do not have greater efficacy than the older tricyclics. Trazadone, a new generation antidepressant, appears to have the least risk of anticholinergic side effects of any of the antidepressants. However, it can potentially cause significant sedation. In addition, it has been found to cause priapism (abnormal, painful, prolonged penile erection) in some males; of course, this would not apply to women who in later life both outnumber men and experience a greater frequency of depression. Amoxapine, another new generation antidepressant, has a small potential to cause tardive dyskinesia, characterized by disturbing muscle movements that may be difficult to reverse. Maprotiline, also a new generation antidepressant, may carry a risk of seizures greater than that for the older tricyclic antidepressants. Because of the relatively low risk of major side effects associated with the use of desipramine and nortripyline for the treatment of depression in the elderly, these two drugs are popular among geriatric psychiatrists.

Monamine Oxidase Inhibitors (MAOIs).
The MAO inhibitors (phenelzine and tranylcypromine) are also quite effective antidepressants in the elderly. Moreover, they tend to have less potential for the anticholinergic, hypotensive, and sedating side effects of the tricyclic antidepressants. The main hesitation in using them is their potential interaction with certain foods or other drugs the patient might be taking, where a risk for high blood pressure develops (Salzman, 1984a). The culprit food substance is tyramine, which is found in various cheeses, yeast extract, caviar, sausage, herring, beef and chicken liver, and large amounts of avocado, chocolate, caffeine, and chianti. Drugs that might also negatively interact with MAO inhibitors causing hypertensive episodes include antihistamines, nonprescription cold and flu medications, dental novocaine dissolved in epinephrine solution, and stimulants. Hence, the diligent monitoring and dietary compliance required on the part of the patient often discourage the physician from using MAOIs. But when the other antidepressants are not effective, the MAO inhibitors sometimes come through.

Electroconvulsive Therapy (ECT).
Considerable confusion and misinformation have surrounded the use of electroconvulsive therapy in general. There is even less awareness of the experience with this modality in the elderly. But modern, modified ECT has been used very safely and quite effectively to treat older depressed patients under certain carefully

specified conditions (Burke, Rubin, Zorumski, & Wetzel, 1987; Sakauye, 1986; Salzman, 1984a). In general, the use of ECT in the elderly is considered for patients (a) when their depression is very severe and other forms of treatment have been ineffective; (b) when the effect of the depression is such that physical health is threatened and coexisting medical problems make the safe use of drugs unlikely, due to the high risk of serious side effects; and (c) in emergencies, as with patients who are very suicidal and not responding to other interventions.

Indeed, ECT is considered the safest approach to severe depression in later life when the risk of side effects of drugs in frail elderly depressives outweighs the potential benefit of these medications. It is certainly safer to use ECT than drugs when the older patient has significant cardiac problems. Its risk of complications is low—typically less than the risk with medications—and with the new techniques in applying it, residual memory problems are unusual. Its primary contraindication is in elderly persons with preexisting increased intracranial pressure. ECT may well be life saving in frail, severely depressed older adults whose worsening weight loss and suicidal impulses require emergency treatment. Drugs often take a month before showing significant therapeutic effect, while results with ECT are much faster, and sometimes almost immediate.

Antipsychotic (Neuroleptic) Drugs and the Elderly

Antipsychotic medications provide good examples of the concepts of trade-offs and the need to individualize drug use in the elderly. Though antipsychotics are similar in efficacy at equivalent dosages, their side effects vary considerably in how likely they are to occur from one drug to the next. They share one group of side effects in common with the tricyclic antidepressants—that of potential anticholinergic side effects, hypotension, and sedation. A different grouping of side effects of antipsychotic drugs is that of *extrapyramidal symptoms,* which include Parkinson-like symptoms, general restlessness (akathisia), a de-energized state (akinesia), and problems of muscle disturbance (dystonic reactions) such as with the "Pisa syndrome" where the patient may tilt to one side.

The antipsychotics that have a high milligram dosage (e.g., one at 100 mg, taken three times a day) are lower in potency; they require a higher dose to reach the desired effect. Hence, they are sometimes referred to as high dose/low potency antipsychotics. The neuroleptics with a low milligram dosage (e.g., one at 1 mg, taken twice a day) are higher in potency; they require a smaller dose to achieve their therapeutic effect. They are sometimes referred to as low dose/high potency antipsychotics. The high dose/low potency antipsychotics are more likely to have the anticholinergic/hypotension/sedation group of side effects; the low dose/high potency

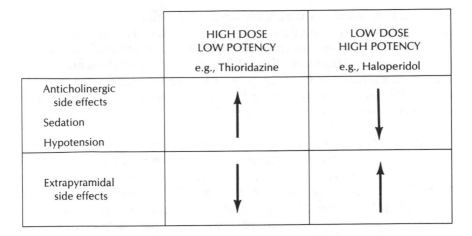

Figure 4.1 Comparative side effect profiles of antipsychotic drug groups.

antipsychotics are more likely to have extrapyramidal side effects. In treating certain elderly psychotic patients who also experience memory problems, the physician might prefer to prescribe a low dose/high potency antipsychotic drug—to reduce the risk of anticholinergic side effects which could aggravate the memory impairment. On the other hand, in treating certain elderly patients who also suffer from a gait disturbance, the doctor might feel it is safer to administer a high dose/low potency neuroleptic agent—to reduce the risk of extrapyramidal symptoms that could further interfere with the difficulty ambulating. The relationship between these two side effect profiles is summarized in Figure 4.1.

More detailed information about antipsychotic medication relevant to their potential use with the elderly is presented in Table A.4 in the Appendix. A number of other potential side effects can occur with any of the neuroleptics, such as tardive dyskinesia alluded to earlier in reference to amoxapine, but the ones included in Table A.4 are the major ones that have been found to *vary* among the different drugs.

Antianxiety and Sleeping Medications for the Elderly

The issue of which antianxiety agent to consider when medication is indicated was alluded to above. More often than not, the physician seeks a short-acting drug that would be metabolized sufficiently fast that it would not build up in the body to become toxic. On the other hand, a longer-acting agent would require fewer dosages, thereby being easier to remember and to monitor in those with memory problems. The primary antianxiety agents used with the elderly are the benzodiazepines which have fewer side effects and better efficacy than other drugs taken to relieve anxiety. Table A.5 in the Appendix lists the major benzodiazepines that are used, along with dosage ranges and the mean elimination half-life of each (the time required for half the amount of the drug to be deactivated or eliminated from the body). Oxazepam, lorazepam, and then alprazolam are commonly prescribed by geriatric psychiatrists.

Sleeping Problems. The antianxiety agents are also considered for treating sleeping problems in the elderly. But insomnia in older adults is a complicated area, where in most cases prescribing sleeping medications is not the best approach and in many not the safest. There are many causes of sleeping difficulties in later life that are more effectively and more safely approached from a nonpharmacologic perspective (Reynolds, Kupfer, & Sewitch, 1984). When sleeping pills are indicated, they are best used briefly to avoid problems of tolerance, dependence, and various potential side effects (Regestein, 1984). Among the safer hypnotics and those less likely to build up in the elderly are triazolam, temazepam, and chloral hydrate. However, these stronger hypnotics (the formal sleeping pills) are often not necessary in the elderly; milder antianxiety agents, such as the short and intermediate acting drugs in Table A.5 of the Appendix, are commonly administered as a bedtime dose for this purpose and frequently preferred by geriatric psychiatrists.

Drugs for Physical Ills That Cause Psychiatric Problems in the Elderly

Early in this chapter, a series of paradigms was described for examining relationships between physical and mental health in the elderly. Though these paradigms were presented more from the perspective of interacting illnesses, they can also be applied to drug use with older adults, as follows:

1. Psychotropic drugs with physical side effects

Example: Amitriptyline   →   Hypotensive episode leading
            (*antidepressant*)   to the patient falling

This paradigm corresponds to much of the above discussion of psychotropic drug use in the elderly, with the choice of drug being governed as much by the goal of avoiding certain somatic side effects as that of achieving therapeutic efficacy for the psychiatric problem.

then, the converse of this paradigm,

2. Drugs to treat physical disorders causing psychiatric side effects

Example: Reserpine   →   Depression
                  (*antihypertensive*)

This example will be elaborated in some detail in Chapter 6. The key point is that not only do psychiatric symptoms in the elderly represent possible side effects of drugs used to treat physical disorders but also that the onset of the symptoms may be delayed and therefore their association with drug use missed. Almost all medications used in the treatment of general medical disorders carry some risk of causing psychiatric symptoms, thus requiring ongoing alertness to this possibility—especially since these symptoms are typically completely reversible (Levenson, 1979).

then, combining the above two paradigms,

3. Problems caused from the interaction of psychotropic medications and drugs for treating physical illness when taken concurrently; these represent drug–drug interactions

Example: Guanethidine (*antihypertensive*) + a tricyclic antidepressant → Decreased effectiveness of guanethidine, leading to elevation in blood pressure

The point illustrated in this example is that either of two drugs alone may not cause disturbing side effects in the elderly, but when taken concurrently they might interact adversely, introducing a new problem. Alcohol, too, can play a major role in adverse reactions with other drugs; its metabolism is also altered in later life, less of it being required to bring on toxic effects. Further examples of drug–drug interactions are myriad, and our understanding of them continues to grow (Salzman, 1984b). That elderly individuals are more likely than younger ones to be on multiple medications explains why the older patient has been one of our greatest sources of new knowledge about the pharmacokinetics of drug–drug interactions in general.

New Clues about Aging

The quest for understanding the intricate dynamics of how pharmacologic agents can control as well as cause psychiatric symptoms is yet another search that leads the scientist to the brain. The brain, after all, is the site both where psychotropic drugs exert their main effects and where many medications for somatic disorders trigger their behavioral side effects. The growth of geriatrics as a formal field of inquiry has catalyzed this exploration in the face of so much medication use by older adults. There is still much to learn about how drugs work, about the fundamental mechanisms through which they operate in influencing the mind. In the process of studying them in the elderly, researchers are certain to uncover further mysteries about the brain—and about how that brain ages. The question of distinguishing between mental disorder and normal mental development in later life will be the focus of the next chapter. Indeed, Part II of this book will concentrate on the problems of disorder and disease in the aging brain.

II

Disorder and Disease in the Aging Brain

5

Differentiating Disorder from the Normal Aging Process in the Brain: Mental Disorders in Later Life

Shakespeare on old age, in *As You Like It:*

Last scene of all,
That ends this strange eventful history
In second childishness and mere oblivion,
Sans teeth, sans eyes, sans taste, sans everything.

Cicero on old age, in *De Senectute*

Intelligence, and reflection, and judgement, reside in old men, and if there had been none of them, no states could exist at all.

As alluded to in Chapter 3 on "Behavior and the Aging Brain," one cannot discern normality if one fails to recognize abnormality. Views vary considerably, as reflected in the observations of Shakespeare and Cicero above, who portray respectively the differential effects of illness and health on the aging process. Perhaps because behavior is difficult to measure, and because it varies so much in different cultures, aberrant behavior is particularly at risk of going unrecognized as abnormal. Again, compare the "second childishness and mere oblivion" and "sans everything" in the "last scene," portrayed by Shakespeare, with the "intelligence, and reflection, and judgement" that "reside in old men," described by Cicero. In the subculture of later life, aberrant behavior may be misinterpreted even more frequently than in the setting of younger adulthood. Behavioral problems in the elderly are commonly misperceived as natural consequences of the aging of the brain.

But people confuse the concept of natural aging brain activity with negative manifestations of what they view as the mind, personality, or behavioral tendencies of an older adult. Also, in the elderly people tend to misperceive behavioral problems more often than somatic symptoms. This probably reflects both the influence of cultural factors and the fact that mental phenomena are more intangible than physical symptoms. Depressed blood pressure in an older person raises concerns about potential falls and fractures. Depressed blood sugar levels sound the alarm about metabolic imbalance. Depressed moods, however, too often fulfill expectations about the fate of older adults. That the major symptoms of Alzheimer's disease are mental and behavioral further explains why for so long people failed to view this disorder as an illness in need of intervention.

Mental disorder and its differentiation from normal mental development in later life will be examined here in some depth. What should become apparent is that aging does not preclude the ability to modify a troubled mind or disturbed behavior in older adults with appropriate interventions. Indeed, in some cases because of advancing years, the course of certain serious illnesses can be more easily modified; a better understanding of such phenomena in the elderly could well help in unlocking further pieces to the puzzle of mental illness at any age.

HISTORY

With the evolution of knowledge in the field of psychiatry has come an increased understanding of the role of several factors that influence the states of mental health and mental illness (Alexander & Selesnick, 1966). We have moved from seeking a magical explanation of madness to the examination of multiple variables along physical and psychosocial axes. These include the impact of biological, psychological, environmental, and familial variables. The interaction of mind, brain, and culture have been examined in efforts to better comprehend mental well-being and mental disorder. Intrapsychic, biomedical, and interpersonal dynamics have all been recognized as playing a part. The approach to treatment has witnessed a similar evolution, from the prehistoric practice of *trepanning* (making a hole in the skull to allow the escape of disease-causing demons) for the seriously disabled, to the more contemporary use of *T*-Groups (sensitivity *T*raining groups) to foster further growth for the well functioning. Present day state-of-the-art talking therapies in combination with pharmacologic treatments have been touted for their dramatic effect on permitting many of the more chronically ill to live in the community as opposed to an institution. Despite this progress in understanding and intervening with mental disorder, much of this knowledge has been unevenly applied for the older person and patient.

Awareness of how this knowledge applies to the elderly, though inadequate, is improving. Comprehensive texts written on the nature and treatment of mental illness in general are doing a better job of integrating information on the elderly (Kaplan & Sadock, 1985; Talbott, Hales, & Yudofsky, 1988). Comprehensive texts focused specifically on the elderly are also being published, reflecting the explosion of new information in this area (Birren & Sloane, 1980; Busse & Blazer, 1980b). Progress has occurred not only in the understanding of mental disorder, but in its treatment as well. A current poll found over 400 types of psychiatric treatment approaches of either a psychosocial or somatic nature, and led to an important publication that attempted to review the state-of-the-art of interventions for mental health problems (Karasu, 1984). While specific issues related to aging are included in that overview, there have been other works devoted solely to treating mental illness in the elderly, through both somatic (Salzman, 1984c) as well as psychosocial (Butler & Lewis, 1977) interventions. Considerable advances have also taken place in the classification and nomenclature for mental disorders, as in *DSM-III-R (Diagnostic and Statistical Manual of Mental Disorders, Third Edition, Revised)* published by the American Psychiatric Association (1987); *DSM-III-R* also reflects recent improvements in the classification of late onset disorders in older adults, as in the case of late onset schizophrenia.

RECOGNIZING SYMPTOMS OF DISORDER IN LATER LIFE

Symptoms of Memory and Concentration Difficulties

When an older person shows symptoms of disorder in later life, they are often missed—several of these symptoms were alluded to in earlier chapters. Significant change in intellectual functioning is fortunately becoming less likely to be dismissed as part of normal aging, given the heightened awareness of Alzheimer's disease. But there continues to be considerable underappreciation of the degree to which depression and anxiety can interfere with cognition. Pseudodementia (to be discussed in Chapter 7) represents an extreme form of this interference. But there are less severe, though still serious forms, as illustrated in the case example that follows.

Case Example: Mrs. Thomas, an 81-year-old woman with an agitated depression (mixed depressive/anxiety state) became even more distraught when she failed the written part of a driver's exam that she was required to take again because of her age. Her self-esteem further plummeted as she thought that on top of everything else her memory and concentration were going as well. It was explained to her that in addition to the dysphoria and agitation she was experiencing, her state of mixed anxiety and depression was interfering with her intellectual skills as well. She was also told that sometimes young healthy college students do poorly on their exams if they too are clinically depressed. Eight weeks later, following a combined approach of psychotherapy and antidepressant medication, she repeated the driving test and easily passed both the written and performance parts.

Change in Sleep Pattern as a Symptom

An older person complaining of sleeping less is commonly assured that this comes with aging—that it is normal, and not to worry. Not necessarily so. Although various sleep studies have found that a reduction in total sleep time can occur in later life, others have not (Feinberg, 1968; Miller & Bartus, 1982). Clinically, it is better to view such change as a group characteristic that does not apply to all individuals, while the reduction which occurs is typically quite gradual. Consequently, sleep changes in the elderly should not be taken for granted, especially if of recent onset. If an older person reports noticeable reduction in sleeping—not just sleeping less at night because of naps during the day—then an evaluation should be done. Apart from potential medical problems of arthritic, urologic, or cardiologic origin, psychiatric disorders can have sleep changes as hallmark symptoms. Early morning awakening may be an important clue pointing to an underlying depression; difficulty falling asleep or restless sleep with frequent awakenings may signal an anxiety disorder.

Change in Sexual Interest or Capacity as Symptom

In Chapter 3, the case of 83-year-old Mr. Obrey vividly illustrates the impact that depression can have upon sexual interest and performance in later life (p. 42). As with changes in sleep pattern, a similar approach should be taken with sexual complaints. One should again be separating group characteristics from the individual case. But even as a group, healthy older men and women with a past history of normal sexual activity and a present situation of sexual opportunity have been found to retain solid interest and capacity for sexual experience. Significant changes, particularly if more recent in onset, deserve a diagnostic work-up. The major areas of focus in an evaluation should include medical/surgical factors, drug side effects, and psychiatric causes. Men are more commonly affected than women by medical and drug influences, since these factors can interfere with erectile and ejaculatory function. More common medical explanations for erectile dysfunction include metabolic and neurologic problems, such as diabetes mellitus, hypothyroidism, malnutrition, and Parkinson's disease. As part of a search for a possible drug role in sexual dysfunction, alcohol should also be considered; not only is alcohol a depressant in higher amounts, thereby negatively influencing sexual interest, it can also interfere with erectile and ejaculatory capacity. Depression or anxiety can affect older men and women alike, in lowering their motivation for romantic involvement and diminishing sexual satisfaction. Regardless of the cause, a substantial number of these problems can be ameliorated or eliminated with proper intervention.

Dread of Death as a Signal of Depression

It was also pointed out in Chapter 3 that dread of death—persisting angst about impending demise in the absence of terminal illness—should be seen as signaling a high likelihood of underlying depression, not a normal rumination of growing old. Even with terminal illness, a variation on this theme of misinterpreting symptoms has been described; in a fairly recent study it was asked, "Is it normal for terminally ill patients to desire death?" Forty-four terminally ill patients, average age 63, were evaluated in terms of whether or not they wished death to come early. The majority (34) were found to have never desired an early death. All 10 who did want to die were found to be suffering from clinical depressive illness; only one of the other 34 was also depressed (Brown, Henteleff, Barakat, & Rowe, 1986). These 11 individuals needed help not only in managing their physical illness, but also their depression, which was exacting a severe emotional toll as well. Of course, most older people are neither dying nor near death, a fact that is commonly overlooked. To the extent that the phenomenology of time and time left is not understood in the case of the elderly, important treatment options might be inappropriately put aside.

Too many clinicians fail to initiate an adequate treatment plan because they are either confused or uneasy about how much time the elderly have left to live. They misinterpret longevity data. Tables that tell us the average life expectancy typically refer to longevity from birth. By age 65, though, one is a survivor, with a new average life expectancy of approximately 15 years for men and 19 for women—intervals that are increasing with the late 20th century medical advances. And these are only averages, with the number of individuals reaching age 100 continuing to grow.

We also have to remember that there is great individual variation in the multimillions of older adults. Mental health treatment needs and opportunities among these millions similarly vary, ranging from the structuring of specialized milieus for protective living to the provision of psychoanalysis. Moreover, many older patients are no less likely than various younger ones to respond to crisis-oriented psychotherapeutic interventions requiring only a few sessions. Brief and effective psychotherapy with the elderly is remarkably more commonplace than is appreciated by the public and practitioners who do not work with older adults.

Psychiatric Symptom as Signal, or Meaning in the Madness

Whereas we recognize symbolism in art and literature, we are less likely to associate it with illness. Freud changed that in psychiatry, when with brilliance he expanded the understanding of the meaning of aberrant behavior and thinking, and led us to an appreciation of psychiatric symptoms as signals of turmoil if not cries for help. Just as unexplained fever alerts one to the possibility of a covert infection, so, too, bizarre behavior can offer a window for catching a glimpse of inner stress. But with the elderly, it is as if one pulls the shades; disturbing changes in a younger person that might raise the specter of schizophrenia desperately in need of intervention, in older adults might be reacted to as annoying eccentricity of aging best ignored or removed for the view of others.

Case Example: A 66-year-old man, Mr. Norton, was discussed in consultation with the new resident manager of an independent-living senior citizens building. She described the man as being very bizarre and provocative. The manager expressed the belief that it would perhaps be better for everyone if the man were not allowed to remain because his behavior so disturbed other residents. For example, when he walked through the building he would be seen spraying air freshener or sprinkling powders on himself, taping pennies to his wrist, and touching a Bible and a bar of soap to his lips. When the manager was asked whether the man actually physically engaged anyone, she only then realized he had not. His disturbance was, in effect, mainly a visual one. No one had been either threatened or harmed by him.

It was suggested to the manager that the bizarre traits of this man were in actuality symptoms, that symptoms are usually signals of underlying problems, and that people under severe stress sometimes indirectly give out messages seeking help in the form of symptoms very varied in nature. It was further suggested that the next time the manager met the man in the building she ask him how he is doing, and she might inform him that she had been concerned about him and wondered if he would like to talk to a doctor who comes to the clinic in the building to help people with their worries and other problems. To her surprise, when she carried out the suggestion, the man accepted her recommendation to see a psychiatrist.

When interviewed, Mr. Norton presented the previously described appearance and demeanor. Not long into the interview the meaning of some of his symptoms became clear. He described horrible hallucinations of smell which he attempted to dilute by applying chemicals and powders to himself, much the way one would use an air freshener to rid bad odors in a room. In addition he expressed considerable guilt about sexual fantasies he had about women other than his wife, who had become bed-bound with illness and physically less able and emotionally less available for lovemaking. Mr. Norton's bizarre way of dealing with this guilt was to attempt to control and cleanse his thoughts with the Bible and the bar of soap, as if his mental images were dirty words on his lips.

Understanding the significance of the pennies taped to Mr. Norton's wrists was considerably more difficult and challenging. It was noticed, however, that whenever he would talk about the terrible odors he smelled, he would rub the pennies. This association suggested the significance of the symptom: Another name for a penny is a *cent*, which in the primary process (magical) thinking to which he had regressed was equated to the homonym *scent*. The patient's primitive symbolic approach to gain control over his olfactory hallucinations was to smother these scents (cents) under tape on his wrists while using the perfume and powders as adjuncts. Meanwhile, comprehensive medical evaluation disclosed no physical or organic basis for his symptoms.

It became apparent that Mr. Norton was suffering from a schizophrenia-like disorder. As best as it could be determined from history obtained from the patient and his family, he did not begin to develop apparent abnormal behavior until his fifties, somewhat later than the more typical onset of schizophrenia before the age of 45. Paradoxically, it is not just with good health in later life that one can witness the tremendous reservoir of energy that is available for a full life course. It can be seen with illness too. This is part of the tragedy of schizophrenia at any age—that so much creative drive can be detoured into disease.

Schizophrenia has come to be regarded as a syndrome, "referring to a condition with a relatively consistent pattern of clinical signs and symptoms which may arise from a number of different initial conditions operating through different mechanisms utilizing different pathways" (Cancro, 1982, pp. 53–54). The origin of schizophrenic illnesses is unknown, though there are considerable research findings to assume that biological, psychological, and social components are all involved (Cancro, 1982).

In an effort to try to better understand some of the deeper psycho-dynamic influences on Mr. Norton's behavior, the following information was eventually pieced together: When he was 11 years of age, Mr. Norton was burned severely in a kerosene fire. He vividly and painfully recalled smelling his own burning flesh along with the subsequent horror and disgust he felt viewing his distorted appearance in the mirror; he felt like a pariah, ashamed of his looks at that young, critical age. Despite his clothes covering most of the burned areas of his body, with his face fortunately only minimally affected, Mr. Norton remained very sensitive about how he looked for many years to follow. Amidst all the normal upheaval of adolescence, Mr. Norton carried the extra burden of a traumatized body image. He became somewhat of a loner, acquiring work as a chef after completing high school. When the last restaurant at which he worked went out of business, he was not able to get a comparably good job, and retired with further damage to his self-esteem. It was apparently during his troubled later life job search that he started to become more symptomatic. His symptoms took on paranoid delusional qualities in combination with the olfactory hallucinations; he felt external forces were manipulating the "putrid" smells about him.

It seems that in the complex and disconcerting nature of the paranoid condition the delusional individual commonly effects a scenario where his perception that those around him are against him gets fueled. If a paranoid person looks threatening—even though not intending to hurt anyone—others may become frightened of the individual and respond in a negative or constraining manner. The paranoid person can then feel "aha, they *are* against me," even though he himself has unconsciously set up the tense interaction. In an extraordinary way, Mr. Norton created a situation where others became appalled by his disturbing visual and odorous presence. He had, with creative pathology so to speak, symbolically re-enacted a situation where he confirmed that others, too, were disgusted by the horrible smells and appearance of his burns, substituting a myriad of sprays and powders for the smells, and the taped pennies, soap, and Bible for the appearance. In his paranoid frame of mind, he knew the "real" reason why people shunned him. There was meaning to his madness.

While the details of these therapeutic discussions were not shared with the manager of the building, early on she was told that this deeply troubled man was tormented by his terribly distressing hallucinations of smell which he tried to control in the ways described above. The aim was to help her understand that he did not will these actions, but was driven to them in desperation. It was described that at times a diabetic who is hypoglycemic can behave as if he were drunk, and that the diabetic's problem was due to a chemical imbalance (of insulin) in the pancreas; in much the same way Mr. Norton's disturbing behavior could be explained by a chemical imbalance (of neurotransmitters) in the brain. Similarly, just as the diabetic's condition is managed by a combination of behavioral (e.g., diet and weight control) and pharmacologic approaches, so, too, behavioral and pharmacologic interventions would likely also benefit Mr. Norton.

She was told that Mr. Norton's problem was likely to be chronic, though capable of being controlled. Her uneasiness about the man, largely due to her fear of the unknown, was replaced by compassion and concern. Through a new understanding of part of the nature of mental illness, her own emotions evolved from fear to curiosity to empathy. She was able to recognize her tenant's problem as a chronic psychosis and came to understand the implication of this diagnosis in terms of the need and impact of long-term treatment.

Over the subsequent twelve-year period the management of the building changed six times. Each new manager "rediscovered" this man, seeing him as an urgent problem who would probably require placement into another setting. In each instance the same consultative intervention was employed, with the same resulting outcome of altered perceptions by the respective managers. Mr. Norton continued to go through a period of exacerbations and remissions with his illness, until his death from prostatic carcinoma at the age of 80.

Several points are illustrated by this case. The significance of psychiatric symptoms should be better appreciated, whether these clinical manifestations are in the form of disturbing behaviors or disturbed thoughts. Symptoms serve as signals, and although they can be difficult to interpret, they typically have a meaning in their own right. The case of Mr. Norton also illustrates that sometimes what happens to someone with a serious mental disorder is not a factor of the natural history of the illness alone, but can be as much determined by the influence of significant others who interact with the ill individual. Significant others can be helping others, or they can be aggravating others.

The different aspects of chronic illness should also be appreciated. The goal of health care is not just to prevent or cure illness, but at times to keep a serious disorder from deteriorating. Mr. Norton's mental illness reached a relative stability; it was the social milieu that was uncertain and caused the biggest challenges to his life course. Moreover, chronic mental illness is often seen differently from chronic physical illness. Physicians, families, friends, know that many severe chronic physical disorders can flare up, causing great distress and management difficulties in getting the illness back under control. But they also understand that flare-ups and remissions can be part of the clinical course of such diseases, that proper treatment will very likely bring even a major exacerbation back under control. Those with labile diabetes and congestive heart failure represent common examples of this phenomenon. Unfortunately, similar understanding about the clinical course of severe chronic mental disorders, as with schizophrenia, is frequently absent among physicians, families, and friends, especially if the patient is elderly. But when these disorders flare up, they, too, can typically be brought back under control, no matter how late in the life cycle. Moreover, with an exacerbation of a physical illness, those close to the patient do not feel that the preceding interval of remission was wasted; they redouble their efforts to help the patient back into remission. Too often with a flare-up of psychiatric symptoms, shoulders shrug and sighs abound from those around the patient, as if previous efforts that brought about a symptom-free period were for nought.

There are important lessons about psychiatric treatment as well in the case of Mr. Norton. Too often false debates are held on which is better in treating mental disorder—drugs or psychoanalysis. Such debates have several flaws: They fail to follow a problem-oriented approach, where different problems require different interventions; they set up false dichotomies, presenting pharmacologic and nonpharmacologic approaches in a competitive rather than a complementary light; they look at supposed therapeutic options narrowly, failing to distinguish for example between psychoanalysis and other forms of psychotherapy; they misleadingly imply that there is always a best approach, as opposed to more than one treatment of choice; they fail to take into consideration individual variation and special circumstances, even in the face of the same clinical syndrome.

In the case of Mr. Norton, treatment combined antipsychotic medication with psychotherapy. Drug treatment for hallucinations or delusions often has a dramatic effect in alleviating these psychotic symptoms. But patient compliance can prove to be a very serious problem with many paranoid individuals. It proved to be a chronic problem with Mr. Norton. Despite a good working relationship with the doctor, he continued to be very resistant to the regular taking of his medication. Interestingly, when his symptoms were particularly severe, causing a significant increase in his level of agitation, he would be more amenable to taking the medicine. The therapeutic relationship was strong enough to gain his cooperation at those times; the continuation of the treatment program over time permitted critical interventions during the periodic crises.

The psychotherapy was essentially supportive in nature. It provided a structure for reality testing and an outlet for Mr. Norton's paranoid concerns. Mr. Norton also derived a sense of personal value from the therapy sessions. Psychotherapy appeared to enhance his self-esteem, as he began to talk about some of his accomplishments in the past and possible new interests in his present situation, with more time gradually being spent on these topics than on his delusions in the discussions.

Masked Symptoms in the Elderly

At the start of the discussion of symptom as signal, an analogy was made between bizarre behavior alerting one to inner stress, just as a fever can signal infection. But sometimes with the elderly patient infection is masked; its usual signs may not be initially produced. For example, a pneumonia can be building in the lungs of a frail aged patient, with none of its hallmark manifestations apparent. The patient may not be coughing; fever may be absent; blood studies may not show an elevated white blood cell count that characterizes so many infections in younger adults. Thus, pneumonia, a major killer in the elderly, can be silent. So, too, depression that can lead to suicide—which is higher in frequency in the elderly than in any other age group—can be silent. Depression in later life can present like an infection without a fever. It can be masked, appearing in an atypical form. Sometimes the clue to depression in an older adult is not in a morose mood or gloomy thoughts expressed by the individual, but in irritating or maladaptive behavior.

Case Example: Mrs. Justin, a 78-year-old woman, came to the outpatient clinic where I have an office, demanding to see a psychiatrist. It would be more accurate to say she stormed into the clinic. The staff was only too pleased to quickly grant her request and escort her to my office. The patient had found herself getting increasingly angry and annoyed, deciding finally to do something about it. It was learned that the woman had suffered severe deterioration in her vision over the past few years, a pathologic process that had not been halted despite extensive opthalmologic intervention and surgery. By the time she sought psychiatric consultation, she was almost totally blind. Not long into the initial interview I became the object of her anger. The patient said she doubted whether I could do anything about her state of mind and that I was probably incompetent anyway. A few minutes later she stomped her cane and exclaimed, "You have confirmed my expectations—you are inept indeed!"

It became apparent that Mrs. Justin was quickly repeating (transferring) in this new relationship what happened in others. She would approach people for help, only then to berate them, driving them away. Her devastating loss of vision had placed her in the position of needing considerable help from others. But this new need to rely on others stirred up a long-standing previously submerged dependency conflict. She had always felt exceedingly uncomfortable in having to depend on someone else. She had always seen herself in the driver's seat of life; anyone with her had to be a passenger—certainly not a guide. Any time Mrs. Justin had found herself in a passive role she would feel uneasy, until she had succeeded in turning things around to assume an active posture. Her situation was a good illustration of the difference between internal (psychological) dependency conflicts and external (practical) dependency needs; it was difficult for her to separate the two. When confronted with practical situations of appropriately having to depend on somebody else because of her blindness, she felt diminished because of her inappropriate psychological need to always do things alone and never depend on others.

This conflict was further reflected in Mrs. Justin's relationship with her family. She had several siblings still living, many of whom encouraged her to visit. Her response, however, was, "Who wants a blind lady?, and besides, I'm not accepting any invitations." Despite her difficulties she continued to display a remarkable degree of energy, initiative, and resourcefulness, though the nature of this activity raised questions.

This 78-year-old blind woman took the bus two nights a week to a course at an inner city university. More unusual was the title of the course: "How to Become a Funeral Parlor Director." She baited me by asking if I knew why she was taking the course. When I bit and asked why, she cuttingly replied, "to perform your funeral."

The tragic loss of vision, "the lights going out," symbolized death to this woman. True to her long-standing pattern of behavior, she was not going to be passive here either, attempting instead to take the offensive. It was as if she felt she was going to get the upper hand on death itself, to gain control over it, by learning how to be a funeral parlor director.

A specific aim of therapy was to help the patient better handle her feelings and behavior in situations where it was appropriate for her to depend on others. The hope was that this would enhance her self-esteem, loss of which had contributed to her depression. The depression, too, would then be helped. Ideally, in this process a considerable amount of energy and resourcefulness would be constructively rechanneled as she worked through the transference issues with the therapist. Over a period of two years Mrs. Justin dealt with her anger and dependency conflict in therapy, and during that time she seemed to come to better terms with them. A turning point had clearly occurred when she finally agreed to visit her family.

This case example demonstrates several points. The importance of looking at aberrant behavior as a symptom is vividly illustrated with Mrs. Justin, and the role of a symptom as a signal of underlying conflict or depression is similarly apparent. Relevant to the preceding chapter, the impact of psychological health on the handling of physical disability can be seen; the converse can be observed as well—i.e., the impact of somatic change on thoughts, mood, and behavior. The place of psychotherapy for the elderly stands out. Above all, the case of Mrs. Justin illustrates that the capacity to deal with crisis and to grow continues throughout the life cycle.

LESSONS FROM SPECIFIC MENTAL DISORDERS IN OLDER ADULTS

Among the many mental disorders that can occur in later life, two in particular will be examined—schizophrenia and depression. Schizophrenia will be looked at in some depth for different reasons. Across the life cycle, it has been seriously understudied, and only more recently has been attracting major new scientific interest (Miller & Cohen, 1987; Natural Advisory Mental Health Council, 1988). It was, for example only in 1987 that late onset schizophrenia was added to official scientific classifications of mental disorders (American Psychiatric Association, 1987). Research on this late onset form of schizophrenia coupled with studies on younger schizophrenics who have grown old with the disorder could well lead to new clues about the better understanding of the illness, independent of age. A focus on schizophrenia in the elderly, in short, provides an important example of the "research on aging as a piece of the puzzle" theme that cuts across this entire book.

Looking at depression in the elderly also illustrates the "piece of the puzzle" theme. In addition, it provides a classic example of how illness in later life can present in atypical ways, offering further understanding as to how a variety of disorders in the elderly ca i be overlooked or misidentified.

SCHIZOPHRENIA IN LATER LIFE

Schizophrenia has historically been very difficult to define, independent of age. It has been even more poorly understood in later life, and yet a focus on schizophrenia in the elderly may well offer important new insights into its nature, cause, treatment, and ultimately prevention, across the life cycle.

Schizophrenia and Paraphrenia (Late Onset Schizophrenia)

Definition of Schizophrenia. In general, one has come to refer to the *schizophrenias* as a "group of illnesses with variable clinical features" (Cancro, 1982). As alluded to above, what causes these illnesses is unknown, though biological, psychological, and social components have all been implicated. Because the illnesses in this group share certain clinical features in common, to differing degrees, they are referred to as the *syndrome of schizophrenia.* Thus, different subtypes of schizophrenia include disorganized type, catatonic type, paranoid type, undifferentiated type, and residual type (American Psychiatric Association, 1987). At some phase of the illness, schizophrenia always involves psychotic experiences such as delusions, hallucinations, or certain other disturbances in thinking; the disturbances are not due to a mood disorder, an organic mental disorder, or substance abuse; there is deterioration from a previous level of functioning; the duration of illness is at least six months (American Psychiatric Association, 1987). Estimates of the prevalence of schizophrenia in the United States range from 0.6 to 3.0% of the population (Babigian, 1985), with similar figures worldwide.

The toll this disorder takes on societies around the world is high; in the United States alone approximately one-fourth of all hospital beds and one-half of the psychiatric beds are occupied by people diagnosed with schizophrenia. Until recently, formal classification manuals had indicated that the onset of schizophrenia occurred before age 45. Increased research on mental illness in the elderly, however, has shown that schizophrenia can have a later life onset in the absence of earlier episodes.

Paraphrenia. Late onset schizophrenia is often referred to as *paraphrenia* in the scientific literature, particularly when paranoid symptoms are prominent (Bridge & Wyatt, 1980a; Bridge & Wyatt, 1980b). Its precise prevalence is not known, though it is significantly less common than early onset schizophrenia.

It was not that schizophrenia-like (schizophreniform) symptoms failed to be observed in the elderly; they were often enough seen but usually dismissed as representing senility, senile dementia, or an organic mental disorder. Such dismissal can have very disadvantageous consequences due to missed treatment opportunities. Treatment of late onset schizophrenia often results in clinical stability or improvement of the condition, while senile dementia typically has a progressive downward clinical course. Interestingly, early historical observations of schizophrenia similarly misperceived the natural history of many *young* people with this disorder. Schizophrenia was initially perceived as having a relentlessly deteriorating course, like that of many dementias. As a result, it was initially named *démence précoce* (dementia of early onset) by the Austrian psychiatrist Morel in 1850 and *dementia praecox* by the great German psychiatrist Kraepelin in 1896.

But Eugene Bleuler, another pioneer in the history of psychiatry and a contemporary of Kraepelin and Freud, recognized in 1911 that dementia praecox did not inevitably lead to deterioration and that its onset was not always associated with adolescence. It was also Bleuler who advanced the view of the illness as a syndrome characterizing a group of disorders rather than a single disease entity (Cancro, 1985b). Bleuler named the syndrome *schizophrenia,* believing the central clinical feature of the illness to be morbid thought processes in the midst of a *split* between thought and mood (Alexander & Selesnick, 1966). A schizophrenic might, for example, be experiencing bizarre thinking or hallucinations that would be accompanied by seeming apathy or even a silly mood; *thoughts* on the patient's mind seem split from the *feelings* conveyed, with both appearing inappropriate. The end result is a high degree of dysfunctional behavior, reflecting inner and causing outer turmoil.

"Dementia Praecox"—Misleading Terminology

The early use of terms like "démence précoce" and "dementia praecox" were confusing enough in describing young schizophrenics. The greater clarity that came in looking at the young did not, however, carry over to the old until much later. While "dementia" had been used descriptively with younger schizophrenics, it became a "diagnosis" in late onset older ones. More recently, the growing recognition of the existence of de novo schizophrenia in later life has resulted in it commonly being referred to as a form of pseudodementia, to the extent it mimics Alzheimer's disease in certain patients. That a significant number of older patients with schizophrenia show varying degrees of clinical improvement over time further distinguishes this disorder from Alzheimer's disease, which always manifests a deteriorating clinical course.

A frequently raised related question is whether older schizophrenics have any different likelihood—greater or lesser—of developing Alzheimer's disease. A detailed review of the scientific literature through 1980 revealed that schizophrenics surviving into later life showed a similar incidence of pathologic brain changes as did mentally healthy old people of comparable age (Post, 1980).

New Views on Schizophrenia from Studies of
Old Schizophrenics

That there has been so much discrepancy in how scientists have viewed schizophrenia in the young makes it less surprising that schizophrenia has been so misunderstood in the old. Beyond missed opportunities for treating various late onset older schizophrenics, opportunities for new insights about the syndrome itself have also been overlooked. By looking at the problem of schizophrenia from a different vantage point, new pieces to its puzzle might be added. Research on the aging schizophrenic can offer such a vantage point. Why is it, for example, that, while the onset of schizophrenia is most common in young adults, certain people can go through so much of the life cycle before becoming symptomatic with the disorder? What is it about these older individuals that caused the onset of the illness to be postponed? Might new clues emerge from study-ing these elderly late onset schizophrenics that could translate into new interventions that could postpone or prevent the earlier onset of the dis-order in vulnerable younger persons?

Moreover, there are likely lessons to be learned about schizophrenia by studying those who have grown old with the disorder. Looking at the natural history of schizophrenia, in general, reports indicate that 10% (Bleuler, 1974) to 23% (Ciompi & Müller, 1976) of those diagnosed with the disorder require permanent or quite prolonged institutionalization, while 20% (Ciompi & Müller, 1976) make lasting recoveries following their first and only attacks. In general, further deterioration of mental and emotional status is no longer seen beyond five years after the onset of psychotic symptoms (Post, 1980).

A major study in Monroe County New York of death rates among schizophrenics found that while mortality was higher among younger schizophrenics (largely due to higher rates of suicide and fatal accidents), it was actually less in older schizophrenics when compared to the general population (Babigian, 1985). Because of advances in the management and treatment of schizophrenia (particularly since the mid-1950s, with the advent of antipsychotic medication), it has been difficult to determine the natural course of the disorder solely as a factor of age. But if one looks at studies prior to the mid-1950s, research showed that schizophrenics surviving into old age tended to experience far less severity in their psy-chotic symptoms, and significantly better social adjustment than at an earlier age (Post, 1980). This has been described in subsequent studies as well, with some referring to the phenomenon as "burnout" (Bridge, Cannon, & Wyatt, 1978).

Why should schizophrenics become less symptomatic and adjust better to their environment in later life? One theory has focused on the role of the neurotransmitter dopamine. A body of literature has mounted which essentially suggests that schizophrenic symptoms occur when the brain responds as if it has an excess of dopamine (Weiner, 1985). This increased dopaminergic *tone* could result from any one of the following: (1) brain neurons could be producing increased amounts of dopamine; (2) brain receptors upon which the dopamine acts could be operating with increased sensitivity to dopamine, such that the same amount of the neurotransmitter is having an exaggerated effect; (3) the effect of one neurotransmitter could be affected by another where, for example, the levels of the neurotransmitters acetylcholine and gamma-aminobutyric acid (GABA) could influence the level of activity of dopamine.

A more recent hypothesis, looking at the reduction in neurotransmitter levels of both dopamine and acetylcholine, has proposed that late onset schizophrenia may represent a relative asynchrony between neurotransmitters; it proposes greater loss of cholinergic than dopaminergic tone—leading to a relative excess in dopamine (Finch, 1985a). Moreover, a related phenomenon is proposed to explain the so-called "burnout" of schizophrenia in those who have grown old with the disorder; based on the dopamine-excess view of the disorder, schizophrenics having a relatively high dopamine tone would—with the normal loss of dopaminergic tone with aging—gradually return toward normal psychological functioning. In either case, by a focus on schizophrenia in general in later life new insights are possible to confirm or revise present understanding and theories about the disorder itself.

The dopaminergic discussion represents, of course, a biological perspective on dynamics observed in schizophrenia with aging. There are also psychosocial views. While examining either biological or psychosocial factors, it is important to keep in mind the background of findings that points to the interaction between them. In my own research on schizophrenia in later life, the sufficiently frequent positive responses of elderly schizophrenics to antipsychotic medications is a reminder of the reported role of altered brain chemistry in the pathophysiology of the disorder and of the high value of drug treatment. Observations from my studies raise psychosocial considerations as well.

Phenomenologic aspects of aging, in the psychosocial arena, appear to have some influence on the course of illness for the patient. For example, part of the acceptance of a person in the community is a factor of how he or she is perceived by others, and these perceptions vary with the age of the individual being viewed. Behavioral symptoms in general are much more likely to be regarded as manifestations of illness in younger adults than older ones; in the latter, they may be dismissed as normal or inevitable concomitants of growing old. On the one hand, this can result in various treatment options for the older person being overlooked. On the other hand, bizarre behavior may be much more easily tolerated in an elderly person than a younger one, resulting in a more accepting social milieu for the older schizophrenic.

It may also be that older schizophrenics experience less threat to their self-esteem in terms of performance expectations. With a peer group more likely to be retired than working, the elderly schizophrenic no longer has the same pressure to perform, and, due to social security, the consequences of not performing are lessened. In a related sense, the older schizophrenic can fit in better, standing out less in terms of task oriented difficulties. Similarly, in face of the likelihood of older persons in general to be living alone (1 in 7 men over age 65 lives alone; 1 in 3 women in this age group lives by herself), social isolation on the part of the schizophrenic in later life appears less in relief. To the extent that psychosocial aspects of schizophrenia in later life do prove to be a significant factor in the altered course of older patients, then a better understanding of these dynamics could translate into improved interventions in the treatment of the disorder independent of age. Advances here might enhance the clinical improvement seen with drug treatment, and perhaps diminish the level and duration of required drug usage; reduced risk of drug side effects would be an added benefit.

In addition to potential new information on biological and psychosocial factors in the schizophrenia, there are opportunities for a greater understanding of genetic and familial considerations as well. There is an increased frequency of schizophrenia in close relatives of those who have the disorder. The results of a large number of studies point to the necessary but not sufficient involvement of a genetic factor; additional factors appear to be necessary to trigger the onset of illness (Cancro, 1985b). In general, the risk of a sibling or a child of a schizophrenic also developing the disorder is on the average 10%, as compared to 0.6–3% for the population as a whole.

What about paraphrenics? There is an increased frequency of schizophrenia in their siblings and children as well; the frequency, though, is less than that of early onset schizophrenics, while greater than that of the general population—somewhere in the middle (Post, 1980). Further research on paraphrenics along this line of inquiry is likely to enhance our understanding of the influence genetic and family factors on schizophrenia per se.

Beyond the implicated genetic base, there is a great need to identify the "necessary" other factors that have been suspected in adding to vulnerability and in precipitating illness. Here, too, studies on paraphrenics can be instructive. A major factor of this nature that has been strongly implicated in late onset schizophrenia is a somatic one—that of sensory impairment. Hearing loss in particular stands out.

The Relationship of Hearing Loss to Paraphrenia

In late onset paranoid disorders, an increased frequency of hearing impairment has been reported (Cooper, Kay, Curry, Garside, & Roth, 1974). Interestingly, the paranoid symptoms in these elderly patients appear to be more closely related to conductive or middle-ear type hearing loss rather than to nerve deafness. Despite the reporting of this relationship, there appears to be little in the scientific literature on modification of psychotic symptomatology as a factor of efforts to ameliorate auditory deficits. Since middle-ear problems may be responsive to one of a number of interventions (e.g., hearing aids, medical or surgical interventions) such approaches should be considered.

Why hearing impairment might have a role in the onset of paraphrenia is not clear. There have been studies, though, that demonstrate the influence of sensory deprivation in the development of very disturbing symptomatology (refer to the case of Mr. Green in Chapter 4, page 58); even young adults can experience difficulty in thought organization as well as hallucinatory and delusional ideation in response to sensory deprivation (Cooper et al., 1974). Given the concept of schizophrenia as a syndrome with an interplay of biological, psychological, and social factors underlying its genesis, hearing loss could be one of those variables which has a precipitating effect on certain vulnerable individuals. Of note is that visual impairment in the elderly has also been implicated as a risk factor in paraphrenia (Post, 1980). The interactions of body and mind—of psyche and soma alluded to in Chapter 4, attract our attention here as well.

The Enigmatic Relationship of Creativity to Schizophrenia

A fascinating study on creativity in schizophrenia revealed that individuals defined as creative had significantly more schizophrenic relatives in their immediate family than did the general population. The study also found that schizophrenic patients had significantly more creative relatives in their immediate family than did the general population (Karlsson, 1970). "These findings suggest that the trait or traits transmitted (genetically) are multipotential and can be a part of high-quality adaptation, as well as play a role in the development of severe illness" (Cancro, 1985b, p. 640). It would be intriguing to explore whether with late onset schizophrenics there is an increased frequency of "late" blooming creativity in their siblings (see Chapter 9 for a discussion of creativity in later life). These elderly paraphrenics might present us with an opportunity not only to find out more about schizophrenia itself, but creativity as well—about illness and human potential.

THE MANY MASKS OF DEPRESSION IN LATER LIFE

Similar to the schizophrenia story, studies of the aging brain in relation to depression expand our understanding of the nature and treatment of depressive disorder in all age groups.

The most important feature of depression in the elderly is that it has many forms (Cohen, 1977). Indeed, it has many masks, making some of its forms difficult to recognize. Like schizophrenia, depression is best regarded as a syndrome, reflecting the common clinical manifestation of a group of disorders (Klerman, 1982). Descriptions of depression go back to antiquity, appearing in biblical, literary, and clinical writings (Alexander & Selesnick, 1966). Throughout, one is struck by the range of efforts to characterize it and to explain its cause.

The term "depression" can be confusing, since it refers to a variety of states—from everyday sadness or blues, to normal grief or bereavement, to clinical depression as a mental disorder. In other words, it represents a *spectrum* of states, where the boundaries can sometimes be fuzzy (U.S. Department of Health and Human Services, 1982). A number of community surveys have reported that approximately 15% of older adults describe significant depressive symptomatology (Blazer, 1986; Blazer, Hughes, & George, 1987). Of these, roughly half are probably suffering from bereavement or a related reactive grief state; the rest appear to have various forms of clinical depression.

The *DSM-III-R* classifies depression under its section on "Mood Disorders" (previously referred to as "Affective Disorders"), and delineates two groupings: (1)*bipolar disorders,* including *bipolar disorder* (e.g., manic-depressive illnesses) and *cyclothymia;* (2) *depressive disorders,* including *major depression* and *dysthymia* (also known as *depressive neurosis*).

In the elderly, the concept of depression becomes even more confusing, but in this confusion lie clues toward greater clarity about depressive disorders regardless of age. In discussions of depression in the elderly, authors often draw upon terminology used to describe disturbances of mood in addition to that of *DSM-III-R*. Findings from geriatric research have, for example, expanded our views on the nature and number of categories of depression. The prevalence of depression in the elderly associated with physical illness and drug side-effects has contributed to the formulation of one of the major classification schemes for distinguishing different types of depression across age groups—*primary* versus *secondary* depressive disorders (Klerman, 1982).

Primary depressive disorders are those occurring in persons who have been well, or whose only prior psychiatric illness was depression. Secondary depressive disorders typically occur in patients who have a physical illness or are experiencing an adverse drug effect. The high frequency of general medical disorders and medication usage among older persons has increased the visibility of secondary depressions. This differentiation has had enormous payoffs in the search for a greater understanding of depression and in approaches to treatment.

Studies on the aging brain have produced findings relevant to theories that attempt to explain biologically what has gone wrong to cause depression, i.e., the nature of the underlying pathology. In the late 1950s a new theory was formulated to explain the genesis of depression. When pharmacological agents for the treatment of depression were introduced in 1957 and soon found to be effective, curiosity abounded as to how these drugs worked. It was theorized that the mechanism of action of these psychotropic compounds could be explained by their effect on certain neurotransmitters in the brain—the biogenic amines, which include the catecholamine neurotransmitter norepinephrine (Cancro, 1985a). The catecholamine hypothesis, simply stated, postulated that the central defect in depression was a depletion in the brain of the neurotransmitter norepinephrine. According to this hypothesis, antidepressant drugs exerted their clinical effect by either increasing the level of norepinephrine or the length of time a given amount of this neurotransmitter would be available to act at brain receptor sites (Schildkraut, 1974). This hypothesis of chemical imbalance, like that focused on acetylcholine in Alzheimer's disease, has an interesting historical antecedent in the postulates of Hippocrates around the 5th century B.C. Hippocrates held that the brain was involved in mental operations and abnormalities, and that mental disorder was the result of imbalances in internal humors (Alexander & Selesnick, 1966; Cancro, 1985a).

As research advanced on the relationship of catecholamine imbalances and depression, new discoveries complicated the picture—among them, certain changes in the aging brain (Veith & Raskind, 1988). One of the brain enzymes that breaks down norepinephrine in the process of metabolism is monamine oxidase (MAO). One of the effective classes of antidepressant drugs is that of the monamine oxidase inhibitors (MAO inhibitors). MAO inhibitors appear to work by inhibiting the action of monamine oxidase, thereby slowing the breakdown rate of norepinephrine as MAO is kept in check. All of this seemed completely consistent with the catecholamine depletion hypothesis of depression.

But studies on the aging brain found that MAO levels increased with aging, while norepinephrine levels diminished (Salzman, 1984a). By the catecholamine theory, then, one might expect to find the elderly as a whole becoming more and more depressed over time. This is not the case. Depression is prevalent enough in the elderly, but most older persons are not depressed. Moreover, there is evidence to suggest that primary depressions may not be more prevalent in older persons than younger ones

(Weissman & Boyd, 1985). Hence, if a reduction in norepinephrine levels coupled with an increase in MAO activity in aging brains does not result in a noticeable increase in the prevalence of depression as would be expected by the basic catecholamine depletion hypothesis, then more must be involved biochemically in the genesis of mood disorders. Research on the elderly suggested that there were further pieces to the puzzle of depression to be discovered by additional studies of the aging brain (Cohen, 1979). Seemingly contradictory findings of this nature have given rise to newer theories, such as the "dysregulation hypothesis of depression," which postulates disruption in mechanisms that regulate the activity rather than the level of neurotransmitters (Siever & Davis, 1985). Another theory of mental dysfunction, alluded to above in aging brain studies on schizophrenia, suggests that asynchrony in the interaction of two or more neurotransmitters is at work in abnormal states of mind (Finch, 1985a).

The Typical Picture of Depression

Persons who are clinically depressed typically manifest a dysphoric mood, a general loss of interest or pleasure in their usual activities, and difficulty with normal functioning. Upon closer inspection, problems can often be identified in five areas: *feelings, thoughts, social behavior, physical status,* and overall level of *functioning.* These five areas are briefly elaborated below:

> *Feelings:* depressed, sad, blue, down in the dumps
> *Thoughts:* expressions of hopelessness, worthlessness, guilt, that nothing is interesting; thoughts of suicide, death; difficulty thinking or concentrating
> *Behavior:* withdrawal from social involvement, less active, irritable
> *Physical:* trouble sleeping, poor appetite, weight loss, fatigue, reduced sex drive
> *Functioning:* difficulty carrying out tasks and normal activities

The above reflect the typical or classical presentation of someone suffering a major episode of depression in the absence of other disorders. Theories vary as to the cause of depression not associated with other illness (i.e., primary depression). With the progress of research, theories that suggest an interplay of biological and psychosocial variables have gained increasing attention (U.S. Department of Health and Human Services, 1981). The interplay of factors is thought to differ among individuals because of their differences in genetic makeup and life history. This "vulnerability" concept has been applied to depression as it has to schizophrenia; individuals are seen as being born with low or high biological susceptibility to depression, having different thresholds for developing the disorder. This could explain why people can go through the same traumatic life experiences, and yet have very different outcomes—some becoming depressed, others not. A corollary to this concept is the idea that whether or not depression develops, depends on the capacity of people and their bodies to adapt to internal and external stressors. Some suggest further that severe, chronic emotional trauma can alter underlying biological systems (nervous and/or neuroendocrine).

As an aggregate, these theories would suggest that the risk of becoming depressed varies with genetic susceptibility and biological status on the one hand, and environmental stressors and coping skills on the other. Hence, one could have a genetic or biological vulnerability to become depressed, but in either the absence of severe enough stressors or the presence of a high level of adaptive coping skills the disorder never results. Attention to age in these studies is increasing and important. Studies on the elderly that show changes in some pattern of the depressive disorder could throw additional light on factors that influence either the aggravation or the alleviation of the disorder. It is thus crucial to study age-associated changes in relation to intervals between depressive episodes, duration and intensity of exacerbations, as well as treatment responses to both biological and psychosocial interventions. The payoff again could be a greater understanding of the causes and treatments for depression across the life cycle.

Meanwhile, the varied masks of depression in the elderly make their appearances as one examines different causes and forms of the disorder in this age group. We will discuss several of these causes and forms below.

Drug-Induced Depression in the Elderly

Given the magnitude of medications used by the elderly, depression as a potential side effect needs to be constantly kept in mind. Unfortunately, many classes of drugs used by older adults can cause depression with varying frequencies (Salzman, 1983). Antihypertensive and antiarrhythmic cardic medications stand out, particularly reserpine, alpha methyldopa, and guanethidine among the former, and propranolol with the latter. Certain diuretics, digitalis, antiparkinsonian drugs, anticancer agents, and corticosteroids have all been implicated. Of course, such side effects are possibilities not probabilities, otherwise the drug would likely not be released.

The risk may be greatest with reserpine, some studies finding the incidence of depression as a side effect of this drug to be 15%. There is another important lesson to be learned about drug side effects by studying the association of depression with reserpine (Cole & Davis, 1975). Examining time of symptom onset, one finds that depression can occur as soon as 1 week or as late as 14 months after starting to take reserpine. Thus the appearance of the side effect can be significantly delayed and, as a result, its cause missed. If after a year has gone by without any trouble, and symptoms of depression only then start to emerge, one might overlook the potential role of the drug; if the drug had been used all that time without side effects, one could be falsely detoured into looking for some other causative factor. The possibility of delayed onsets of drug side effects, therefore, should always be considered in seeking the cause of depression in the elderly—indeed, in general.

Depression in Association with Medical and Neurological Illnesses

The manifestations of a major general medical or neurological illness may mask a coexisting or secondary depression in the elderly. When a disorder is seen as being severe to begin with, coexisting problems may be perceived as being yet further manifestations of the primary disorder, without a proper problem-oriented treatment plan being implemented. Stroke and Parkinson's disease—both largely disorders of later life—are commonly associated with depression; various studies have found the prevalence of depression in each case to exceed 40% (Folstein, Maiberger, & McHugh, 1977; Mayeux, Stern, Rosen et al., 1981; Robinson & Forrester, 1987). Both stroke and Parkinson's disease have clinical features that provide alternative explanations for depressive symptomatology, allowing the latter to be overlooked. For example, both stroke and Parkinson's disease can cause altered facial expressions, thereby masking the sad looks of a depressed patient. Given the high prevalence of depression in certain neurological and general medical disorders in older adults, the burden should be as much on ruling depression out than on ruling it in.

Vague Physical Decline Masking Depression

Vague physical decline in later life does not always point to the natural course of physiologic aging or the subtle progression of underlying physical illness. One commonly sees with the elderly the impact of psychosocial factors aggravating medical problems, at times precipitating a latent physical disorder. The nature and rate of physiologic change in later life can, under the influence of depression, reflect the will to live or die. What may on the surface, for example, appear to be deterioration of overall health due to congestive heart failure may underneath represent despair on the part of the patient, followed by a feeling of giving up and an act of self-termination of medication; the covert suicidal behavior could be missed.

Masked depression in the elderly can lead to insidious loss of appetite with poor food and fluid intake, resulting in dehydration, anemia, or vitamin deficiency, mimicking physical frailty or even the cognitive decline seen in early Alzheimer's disease. This is especially so in those at a very advanced age where so much change is too readily dismissed as the inevitable consequence of growing old. In short, change in general health status in later life should be approached first with clinical questions rather than compassionate resignation. That suicides continue to occur most often in the elderly—especially in white males over 75—should punctuate the need for diligence in searching for underlying depression in older adults (Blazer, Bachar, & Manton, 1986). Depression, after all, is a major risk factor for suicide.

Multiple Somatic Complaints as Maskers of Depression

Concerns about one's body have been found to be quite high in studies of depressed older persons. In one study of 152 depressed patients over age 60, somatic concerns were found in 65.7% of the men and 62% of the women (Busse & Blazer, 1980a). While physical symptoms and multiple somatic complaints in the elderly require diligent medical attention, part of that attention should include a search for underlying psychogenic factors. If psychosocial factors are suspected, one should not suggest to the patient that it may be all in his or her head—not if a follow-up visit is desired. Here, too, challenging a person's symptoms is usually counterproductive, with the patient losing confidence in the clinician. Regardless of the cause of these complaints, whether physical or psychological, the distress to the patient is strongly felt. The distress should be acknowledged, but a diagnosis avoided. These patients probably have been evaluated by different physicians and know that an explanation for their symptoms has been elusive. One should continue from there, acknowledging the complexity of the patient's situation, indicating the need to get a better understanding of the person as a whole. In the process, and through follow-up visits, the focus of the discussion has a chance to shift from the somatic to the psychosocial.

In time, the meaning of the patient's symptoms may become apparent. Depression can lead to social withdrawal or isolation, a greater risk in the elderly; in the process, energy that was invested in interpersonal interactions can be turned inward, with an exaggerated focus on oneself, allowing every ache and pain to become magnified. Older people with fewer friends and family may feel in a bind if they get into conflicts; they may have trouble dealing with their rage, fearing they will drive away the few that remain if they express their true feelings, turning that anger inward where it shows up as physical instead of emotional pain. The elderly are at increased risks for diverse losses (e.g., loss of spouse, economic status, physical health, overall independence); losses can lead to diminished self-esteem and depression, to a disturbing sense of lost "control" of one's life in general, resulting in physical symptoms that represent maladaptive efforts to signal for help, gain attention, or "control" others.

The goal of intervention is to facilitate the shift of focus from the specific complaints to the factors that caused the stress. The aim is to help the patient come to terms with the underlying conflict, and to develop new strategies in attempting to deal with it.

Pseudodementia and Alzheimer's Disease and Depression

As will be discussed in Chapter 7 on the treatment of Alzheimer's disease, depression in relation to cognitive impairment needs to be considered from two perspectives. When considering depression in the differential diagnosis of dementia the clinician must not only consider the possible role of depression alone, but depression in combination with dementia. By itself, depression could be causing a "pseudodementia"; combined with dementia, depression could be causing an "excess disability" state. In either case, the diagnosis and treatment of depression would result in clinical improvement for the elderly patient. The case of Mrs. Thomas on page 80 (this chapter) illustrates the part depression can play in pseudodementia, while the case of Professor Janof on page 153 (Chapter 7) shows the involvement of depression in excess disability.

Suicide in the Elderly and Depression

Though suicides are carried out for different reasons, depression is among the most common. National data show that suicide rates among those 18–24 years of age increased significantly from 1970 to 1980. Nonetheless, the highest suicide rates in the United States continue to be found among those 65 and older (Blazer et al., 1986; Manton, Blazer, & Woodbury, 1987). The differences are most striking among white males. Suicide is nearly 25% more common among white males aged 65–74 as compared to those aged 18–24; it is over 70% more common among white males aged 75–84 as compared to those aged 18–24. Among other explanations for higher suicide rates in older adults, the possibility of widowhood as an important risk factor has also been raised.

While depression and widowhood have a high prevalence among the elderly, one cannot point to age-associated factors alone in attempts to explain differences in suicide rates. Comparing rates among white females as a factor of age, for example, one finds that in 1970 suicide was 32% higher among white females aged 75–84 as compared to those aged 18–24; in 1980, suicide was 36% more common in the younger group as compared to the older one. Hence, even the role of widowhood in suicide is questionable—with the role of widowerhood less clear. In addition to age differences, cohort groups are being scrutinized (population groups that grew up during different historical periods, such as the youth of the 1920s as contrasted to the youth of the 1940s). Different cohort groups appear to have different suicide rates in old age as well as during other phases in the life cycle.

By examining data as a factor of *age* across cohort groups, we are gaining new clues about the disturbing and perplexing problem of suicide in all age groups. One investigator, for example, pointed out that throughout the 20th century in America suicide rates among 15- to 24-year-olds have been high when the percentage of that group in the general population has been high (Hendin, 1982). Altered opportunities for achievement, recognition, employment, and associated alienation are being looked at as dynamics affected by cohort group densities that might be additionally involved in suicide.

Best Face Forward as a Masker of Depression

Depression in the elderly may be atypical in other ways. It may hide behind a smiling face. Certain older individuals have a sufficiently significant number of dysphoric days, spanning a lengthy enough period of time, to have a major effect on the quality of their lives, if not an important influence on their overall level of functioning. But when they are visited by someone or go for a medical checkup, they frequently put their best face forward. Often these individuals live alone, their mood affected by a feeling of isolation. The social or medical contact is emotionally uplifting—the anticipation, experience, and aftermath of the meeting putting the person in a positive frame of mind. Moreover, the older person's uplifted mood during such interchanges can color recall of recent distress, making the prior dysphoria seem no longer an issue. Rather than the individual trying to cover up troubling feelings, it may be more a matter of one feeling over the hump under the influence of the moment. If the clinician does not probe, the problem may be missed. Part of a good checkup is probing.

Though this clinical scenario resembles the description of a dysthymic disorder (depressive neurosis) where a relatively persistent depression may be intermittently broken through by periods of normal mood lasting a few days to a few weeks, there are differences. The ability of the patient to pull out of the dysphoric mood seems greater in the "atypical depression" of the elderly, thereby making it more difficult to diagnose, and easier to overlook. At the same time, this form of depression in the elderly appears especially responsive to supportive interventions.

OTHER MENTAL DISORDERS OF OLDER ADULTS

There are a number of other mental and behavioral disorders suffered by older adults. Not all will be discussed here. Among them, anxiety disorders, manic-depressive (bipolar) disorder, personality disorders, alcohol use disorders, and delirium will be only briefly touched on.

Like depression, *anxiety* refers to a spectrum of states. The manifestations of anxiety can be seen in conditions ranging from normal fear reactions to severe phobic disorders (Verwoerdt, 1980). Because of the physical symptoms that can accompany the psychological distress of anxiety, and because of the manifestation of an anxiety-like clinical picture with various medical illnesses, anxiety in the elderly has been discussed in Chapter 4, which focuses on interrelationships between physical and mental phenomena in older adults.

For related reasons, problems associated with alcohol use (Hartford & Samorajski, 1984; Maddox, Robins, & Rosenberg, 1984) were also discussed in Chapter 4. The literature of both science and the humanities is instructive here as well. Studies point to groups of individuals who as they age appear to diminish or terminate their intake of alcohol (Holzer et al., 1984). The literary work considered to be the first modern short story portrays one such case; *Rip Van Winkle,* written in 1819 by Washington Irving, is at one level the story of a man who in effect sleeps away his early adulthood with a drinking problem, but later overcomes the problem and emerges with new status in his village. A better understanding of what enables various aging individuals to overcome their drinking problems may lead to new insights into the treatment or prevention of alcohol problems in general.

Delirium in the elderly (also referred to as "acute confusional states" and "transient cognitive disorders") typically reflects the influence of physical illness or drug intoxication on the aging brain; it may be potentially life threatening but also potentially reversible (Lipowski, 1983). The case of Mrs. LaRue in Chapter 4 (page 52) illustrates how a constellation of general medical problems, aggravated by psychosocial stress, can bring on an acute confusional state.

More can be said about the need for further study of manic-depressive illness in the elderly than about a literature of any real depth on it (Roth, 1955; Zung, 1980). Of note, though, in that literature, is the emphasis on the atypical appearance of manic episodes in the elderly, where marked agitation may more likely be seen than the typical overactivity of mania in younger adults; similarly, obsessive thought patterns may be more characteristic of older manics than the flight of ideas observed in younger ones. Accurate diagnosis is important, since older manics like younger ones respond to treatment with lithium. Just as the study of the varied manifestations of schizophrenia in later life will likely add new clues to understanding the basic disorder itself, the same should apply to studies on manic-depressive illness in the elderly. We have with these geriatric patients another opportunity to gain a new window on a major disorder of younger adults.

On the topic of personality disorders in later life, the scientific literature is once again sparse, despite a review of various epidemiological studies suggesting that 2.8% to 11% of older adults manifest these conditions (LaRue, Dessonville, & Jarvik, 1985; Sadavoy & Leszcz, 1987). The personality disorder in the elderly perhaps most addressed by clinicians is that where the patient manifests problems with dependency; this applies to patients in both community and nursing home settings. Dependency issues can be quite complicated in older patients—witness the case of Mrs. Justin in this chapter (page 87). From a different perspective, given the frequency of dependency conflicts among aged persons, clinical experience with this patient population puts the clinician in good shape for dealing with dependency problems in general, which are so common across the life cycle. We will return to the theme of what the practitioner can learn from the older patient in the discussion to follow on psychotherapy and the elderly.

DIFFERENTIATING DISORDER FROM DEVELOPMENT IN THE AGING BRAIN

It is not only through a study of illness in later life that one can gain new understanding about disorders in earlier phases of the life cycle. Research on treatment approaches with the elderly can also potentially help expand our views of how to approach diseases across generations. In general, when we find a treatment that works, a search for its mechanism of action might also lead us to the mechanism of illness. Certainly this is true with drugs, and is illustrated with the discovery of antidepressants which led in turn to the biogenic amine hypothesis of depression. Studies of interventions, moreover, can lead to new insights about health and development apart from disorder.

The use of psychotherapy with the elderly, for example, challenges the therapist to better comprehend developmental issues in later life, so that therapeutic technique can best be matched with cognitive and emotional considerations arising at that stage of the life cycle. That the richness of these opportunities with older patients has been overlooked reflects again on the difficulty in recognizing the capacity for change and growth in old age. To be sure, both psychotherapy and drug treatments can activate those capacities in the elderly. However, because of the many physiologic considerations in the use of psychotropic medications, this type of intervention has already been discussed in Chapter 4. Here, we will focus on what we may expect to learn and achieve through psychotherapeutic approaches with the elderly.

There are, of course, other mental health treatment modalities beyond psychotherapy and psychopharmacology. These, along with those mental disorders in the elderly not mentioned here, can be reviewed in various textbook chapters (Cohen & Eisdorfer, 1985; LaRue et al., 1985) and major edited works (Birren & Sloane, 1980; Busse & Blazer, 1980b) on mental health and aging.

PSYCHOTHERAPY AND THE ELDERLY

Past discussions of the role and efficacy of psychotherapy with older people have been replete with misinformation and stereotyping. Research on and success with psychotherapy and the elderly has been well documented since the first quarter of the 20th century (Abraham, 1979; Berezin, 1972; Blum & Tross, 1980; Cohen, 1981; Gallagher & Thompson, 1983; Rechtschaffen, 1959). But the doubters largely held the day until the fourth quarter of this century. Freud started as a doubter. In 1905 he wrote that "the age of patients has this much importance in determining their fitness for psychoanalytic treatment, that on the one hand, near or above the age of 50 the elasticity of the mental processes, on which treatment depends, is as a rule lacking—old people are no longer educable—and, on the other hand, the mass of material to be dealt with would prolong the duration of treatment indefinitely" (Freud, 1978, p. 264).

It is ironical that Freud wrote this as he was nearing his 50th birthday, a period in his own life reflecting considerable elasticity and educability. Ironic, too, is that Freud's regard of "the greatest masterpiece of all time" was a work done by an aging playwright in his eighth decade (Jones, 1957). Sophocles was 71 when he wrote *Oedipus Rex,* the drama that was probably perceived by Freud as a brilliant literary validation of his cornerstone concept of the "oedipus complex" in his then pioneering psychoanalytic theory. Similarly, Dostoevsky was approaching his 60th birthday when he completed *The Brothers Karamasov,* a narrative Freud referred to as the "greatest novel ever written," dealing with the "same theme" as *Oedipus Rex* (Jones, 1957). Dostoevsky died the next year. Could it have been that the "mass of material," as Freud referred to it, that these aging authors had to deal with served to permit them, rather than restrict them, to achieve their great works, their great insights? Could it have been that age-related dynamics allowed certain perspectives to more easily come to mind?

Fifteen years after Freud's reflections on psychoanaylsis for the elderly, Karl Abraham, another giant in the early psychoanalytic movement, expressed a different view in his classic 1919 paper on the "Applicability of Psycho-Analytic Treatment to Patients at an Advanced Age" (Abraham, 1979). Abraham wrote:

> At first it was only after some hesitation that I undertook cases of this kind. But I was more than once urged to make the attempt by patients themselves who had been treated unsuccessfully elsewhere. And I was, moreover, confident that if I could not cure the patients, I could at least give them a deeper and better understanding of their trouble than a physician untrained in psychoanalysis could. To my surprise a considerable number of them reacted very favorably to the treatment. I might add that I count some of those cures as among my most successful results.

Despite Abraham's success and reports, decades of doubts about the place and potential benefit of psychotherapy for older adults persisted. Santayana's observation (paraphrased from Beck, 1980, p. 703) that "those who ignore history are doomed to repeat its mistakes" could not have been more relevant to those who maintained ignorance about major psychiatric success in work with the elderly reported for well over half a century.

The Older Person as Patient: Paradoxes and Possibilities

To the unfamiliar, the interesting possibilities in psychotherapeutic work with older adults may seem like paradoxes. Stereotyped views of aging and the elderly short-circuit clinical considerations. Already alluded to is the part played by misinformation about "time" left and the capacity for "change" in later life—about the seeming paradox around the juxtaposition of the two delightfully captured by Somerset Maugham's description of the elder Cato taking up Greek at the age of 80. Maugham, initially surprised, later reflected that "old age is ready to undertake tasks that youth shirked because they would take too long." Indeed, the capacity for change in later life has been well illustrated from the time of Cato to that of Colonel Sanders. The matter of time left in later life has also been discussed, and here, too, there is interesting historical perspective. For example, in Rome, during the period of the Roman Empire, because of death associated with childbirth, disease, famine, and war, average longevity was only 22 years (Hendricks & Hendricks, 1977). Meanwhile, in contemporary America, at age 65, average longevity is approaching 20 years, with those over 85 representing the fastest growing part of the population. Time and change considerations, therefore, make the case *for* rather than *against* psychotherapy for the elderly. One might say that "they are finally ready to do it right," with more time and fewer distractions toward that goal. Most of the case examples presented throughout this book reflect these points.

There are other areas highly relevant to psychotherapeutic considerations for older adults where we might view later life phenomena and come up with different interpretations. Consider, for example, discussions about apparent repetition of ideas, themes, and behaviors in aging individuals. Metaphorically, one might ask to what extent such apparent repetition reflects a rerun, to what extent an attempted remake (Cohen, 1985a). Whereas a rerun might be regarded in the category of reminiscence, a remake attempt could reflect new material—an effort drawing upon new strategies. People do not make patronizing judgments about film producers or playwrights who attempt remakes of classical myths and stories. Older persons, too, may revisit earlier themes or chapters from their own lives and try them out with a new twist as part of the ongoing process of human growth and development throughout the life cycle.

There are many memories and insights of older people for which we are very appreciative that they have not "gone with the wind." Such oral histories are part of a family's heritage. This perspective deserves consideration in the face of disparaging views on reminiscence, as if reflecting on one's past was merely a compensatory act for something lost from the past, rather than a transmission or sharing of something important from that past. But returning to one's past may at times be more than a life review; it may represent an attempt at a new integration as the older person continues to explore life's meaning as well as his or her own raison d'être.

Related to this discussion is the question as to whether the elderly "slow up" or "slow down." The difference may be more than semantic. Slowing down has a pejorative connotation, while slowing up suggests something of more neutral value. Such concerns relate to analogies between aging and entropy—a continuation of century-old thermodynamic and mechanistic frameworks for viewing psychodynamic phenomena. Prevailing concepts in physics have not uncommonly influenced concurrent formulations in psychology. Even within a mechanistic framework, however, there are alternative analogies pertaining to alternative views on psychodynamic changes experienced by the elderly.

Moving from 19th century engines to 20th century satellites, for example, consider a spaceship which early in its course launches into its journey with tremendous thrust and great force as required to get going on its desired course. Eventually, it releases its boosters, and "slows up" its thrust, as less force is necessary to maintain its journey on course. The analogy to one's journey through the life course is no doubt apparent. Do we need the same booster strength to keep us on an emotionally stable life course with aging, or does a certain positive psychological momentum build up for the majority of older adults? There is varied evidence to suggest the latter, as with those who display less aggressiveness, competitiveness, or impulsivity, as they handle stress more easily in later life. From my longitudinal research on those with psychiatric diagnoses, adaptive changes here, too, are apparent with certain types of problems; with aging there are those whose ulcers settle down, persons who had been anxious in the company of others (social phobics) who become socially more at ease, and schizophrenics whose tormenting symptoms burn out.

There is another area that invites an expanded view. Too often change in later life is scrutinized for evidence of loss or decline, rather than being searched for traces of new strategies. William Carlos Williams, the physician/poet, has written eloquently on this issue. In his sixties, Williams suffered a stroke, leaving him physically but not mentally impaired. He then turned full time to the writing of verse, waxing wisely about an "old age which adds as it takes away" (Foy, 1979). From a psychodynamic vantage point, disproportionate emphasis has been placed on what old age "takes away." A comment by Bertrand Russell (1960) at age 87 also illustrates society's tendency to dwell on perceived losses as opposed to perceived opportunities in later life: "They tell me that if only I took drugs my hair would turn black again. I'm not sure that I should like that because I find that the whiter my hair becomes the more ready people are to believe what I say." The clinical literature is replete with well-articulated allusions to later life as a "season of loss" (Berezin, 1963) or a "crisis in slow motion" (Pfeiffer, 1976), with postulates of a "depletion hypothesis" (Cath, 1966) or a "disengagement theory" (Cumming & Henry, 1961) in efforts to explain decrement naturalistically. Researchers and clinicians have for the most part only just begun to look at what old age adds, an orientation with potentially major ramifications for the psychotherapeutic process. This topic will be elaborated in considerable detail in the discussion of creativity with aging in Chapter 9, where concepts like "emergentive originality" will be discussed—Taylor's (1974) view of a later life capacity to create original or essentially new ideas.

Up until the present cohort group of older adults we have largely not had a true opportunity to see what normal aging can be like. Obscuring the potentialities of normal aging has been a social climate of inordinate stresses emanating from inadequately developed socialization networks for the post-retirement population, sparse high quality age-oriented

activities, housing dilemmas, financial problems, transportation difficulties, and the like. We have not really seen what the true possibilities
for later life can be, free from these external stressors. Compounding the
shortcomings in the social system has been a lack of familiarity with new
opportunities for improved treatments and preventive interventions for
illness. In short, the combination of excessive social stress and illness has
impeded opportunities for further inner growth and development that
can accompany normal aging. Psychotherapy has been too long overlooked as a viable pathway through some of these impediments for many
older persons.

Process and Technique in Psychotherapy with the Aging

The issues that surround process and technique in psychotherapy with the
elderly are many and rich. They range from "transference" (unconscious
tendency of a person to assign to others in the present and immediate
environment those feelings and attitudes originally linked with significant
figures earlier in the person's life) and "countertransference" (conscious or
unconscious emotional response of the therapist to the patient) considerations to those of resistance and insight, among others (Gelfand, 1980).
Berezin reminds the therapist that "transference by definition is unreality;
it is unconscious and is not time-oriented. In this sense it is also consistent
with the concept of timelessness. In psychotherapy, transference reactions
do not follow chronological calendar considerations" (Berezin, 1972,
p. 1487). This is not to say that the age of the patient or the age of the
therapist has no dynamic influence on transference or countertransference
phenomena. The point is that age may or may not make a difference. The
older patient may respond as if the therapist were his or her child, sibling,
or parent. Similarly, the therapist may find himself or herself relating to
one older patient as if the person were "an elder," to another in a parental
mode, and sometimes both ways at different times with the same patient.

A poignant illustration of a shifting transference occurred in my work
with Mrs. Crawford, an 80-year-old childless widow, struggling with
depression, and intermittently troubled over a period of decades by disturbing dreams that re-enacted unresolved conflict with her father
(Chapter 7, page 158):

> During the first few months of therapy the patient would fre-
> quently say something to the effect that I was like a son to her. That
> Mrs. Crawford had been childless not by choice suggested that this
> transference served an important compensatory function. As ther-
> apy progressed, the transference changed. She began to talk more
> about relationships with men and took noticeably more care in her

appearance around me. For one of our sessions she brought a photograph of herself in her twenties, in a 9 × 12 in. frame designed to stand on a table. The clinic where we met had but a small room for us, furnished with a desk and chair for the doctor, and a chair beside the desk for the patient. While talking about the photograph, she placed it on the desk in such a manner that it partially blocked my view of her. As I looked at her, I saw the picture instead of her face. It appeared that she was trying to get me to see her physically as a younger woman. The transference had shifted, as if in her unspoken fantasy we were lovers of a common generation.

The next session led to her looking back at the men she had been attracted to during her marriage, relationships that she recalled were accompanied by anxiety, moodiness, and bad dreams. An association followed where she wondered in retrospect whether the distrustful feelings with which her father had hurt her in adolescence had come back to haunt her when she fantasized about affairs while married. She then asked me how I viewed a married woman having thoughts about other men. I thought to myself that the transference had again changed, that she was attempting to place me into a paternal role. In this new transference, she was confronting the conflict with her father, having a chance to finally resolve it in her ninth decade.

Apart from transference phenomena, this case again illustrates the capacity to confront conflict, gain insight, and resolve emotional struggles, despite—or perhaps because of—advanced age. It should also be pointed out that the role of psychotherapy was not incidental.

Older patients can take you by surprise and turn the tables just like younger ones. Typically the transference is involved. One such memorable episode occurred with Mrs. Sherman.

Case Example: Mrs. Sherman was an 81-year-old diabetic widow who I was asked to see because of the feared consequences of a severe grief reaction that had entered its fourth week, marked by deep sadness, social withdrawal, a pronounced loss of appetite, and growing weakness. Due to the patient's diabetes which required insulin to control, the public health nurse was quite concerned that the appetite disturbance might lead to a medical crisis.

Upon further evaluation it was learned that Mrs. Sherman's 34-year-old (and favorite) grandson had been very recently brutally murdered in a robbery. The patient had just been visited by him two days before his death. The rest of her history and workup revealed no recent change in her overall medical status and no previous psychiatric history other than a prolonged period of bereavement following the death of her husband 12 years earlier. Diagnostically, it appeared that she was experiencing an adjustment disorder with a depressed mood of serious magnitude. Psychotherapy was carried out during weekly home visits.

Mrs. Sherman was very receptive to my visits, and by the third week her depression was lifting with appetite returning. Each new session found her increasingly more able to move the discussion away from the death of her grandson to a description of her own life. It became apparent both from her presence and her history that she had provided great cohesiveness to her extended family, that among her friends and relatives she was a much admired elder. There was a feeling of great warmth and inner strength about her, making it easy to understand why she was so influential on her family. That she was physically a diminutive woman, only five feet tall and under a hundred pounds, made her emotional strength all the more impressive.

I felt that her strongly positive reaction to me—her almost immediate positive transference—was partly a factor of my being about the same age as her grandson at that time. Nonetheless, as Mrs. Sherman's mood improved and her confidence came back, she seemed to be starting to feel somewhat uncomfortable finding herself in a receiving role rather than her usual giving posture. This aspect of the transference dramatically culminated at the end of one of our visits. As I got up to leave, walking toward the door, she sprung up and moved quickly behind me. The next thing I knew she was pulling up my pants from the rear. Taken quite by surprise I turned with a puzzled look on my face, but before I could utter a word she explained with a very satisfied grin of one in command, "Your pants were sagging; you really should pull them up, you know." She took immense pleasure at that moment, looking as if she were back in her more familiar role of the family matriarch. No comment was required; I smiled, and said I would see her next time.

By the eighth week of supportive psychotherapy, Mrs. Sherman was back to her regular self. We wound up treatment on the tenth visit.

The development of a strong, positive transference helped mobilize the patient's emotional energy, enabling her to more quickly pull out of her depression. The case of Mrs. Sherman also serves as an important reminder that brief psychotherapy can be a very effective treatment modality for the elderly; the opportunity for crisis intervention and the efficacy of short-term interventions are far more common than most realize in this age group. We see again that challenge, unpredictability, and rebound are not monopolies of younger patients. From a different vantage point, this case shows that in older patients, like younger ones, change is not always dependent on insight.

What about insight in the elderly? Insight is often discussed in relation to resistance. Grotjahn pointed out that "it looks as if resistance against unpleasant insight is frequently lessened in old age. Demands of reality which in younger people are considered narcissistic threats may finally become acceptable . . . . It seems as if, more or less, suddenly resistance is weakened and insight occurs just because it is high time" (Grotjahn, 1955, p. 420). Indeed it was a 71-year-old who with insight first wrote about Oedipus.

Whereas the nature of resistance and insight relate to the patient's influence on the process of psychotherapy, the practioner brings to bear his orientation and technique. One of the more written about techniques is that of the life review. Butler described the life review approach as a therapeutic use of reminiscing to resolve, reorganize, and reintegrate what is troubling or preoccupying the patient. It is an effort to facilitate the capacity of older people to reconcile or come to better terms with the meaning of their lives (Butler, 1963). Other clinicians and researchers have emphasized the importance of questioning when and for whom to use the life review technique. They point out that some older people will look at past life experiences not as they have been, but as they might have been, and in the process experience guilt and a profound sense of loss. Thus, the existence of a technique is not enough. The therapist must have the necessary understanding and ability to use it properly. Weinberg addressed this concern when he wrote about "adding insight to injury" (Weinberg, 1976). An observation (author's paraphrase) by H.L. Mencken also seems applicable: "For every complicated problem, there is a simple solution; and that simple solution always fails." Psychotherapy with the elderly—its indication, form, and duration—is no less complicated than psychotherapy with younger adults. At the same time, its efficacy among older patients is no less impressive.

Working with Older Patients: Positive Effects on the Therapist

Not uncommonly, therapists working for the first time with older patients are surprised to discover how satisfying the experience can be. That older patients are often more realistic in their treatment objectives and grateful even for small changes in therapy are pleasant realizations. Victims themselves of negative stereotypes of old age, many elderly individuals may not initially expect much to happen in therapy, so when progress does occur, a profound sense of satisfaction can be shared. Psychotherapeutic progress is the rule rather than the exception in this age group.

Moreover, therapists typically gain new information about themselves in conducting psychotherapy with older patients. Whenever one works with any new age group—whether children, adolescents, young adults, the middle aged, or older adults—opportunities arise to see oneself in a new light. Different patients challenge the therapist in different ways, enabling the clinician to gain new glimpses of countertransference phenomena, and to obtain a better sense of one's technical strengths and weaknesses. These new personal insights will benefit the therapist in his or her work with all age groups.

Working with those at an advanced age may, in addition, offer the therapist a unique opportunity to look back in time with the patient at the course of early life conflicts and problems across the life cycle, to examine in one person the interplay of development and disorder over a period of decades. One has the remarkable chance to have a 60-, 70-, even 80-year retrospective follow-up of interactions among psychological, biological, and social changes in the same individual—an extraordinary panorama possible only with older patients. Psychotherapy with the elderly, in short, adds to the therapist's general education; it expands ones understanding of illness and the human condition.

6

Alzheimer's Disease: Modern Medicine's Great Mystery

Alzheimer's disease has emerged as one of the great mysteries in modern day medicine—a devastating disorder with increasing but diverse clues that are taking us down different pathways in the search for cause. The quest to unravel this mystery has taken investigators from the corners of the globe to the depths of the brain (Cohen, 1987; Katzman, 1983; Katzman, Terry, & Bick, 1978; Reisberg, 1983; 1986; Wurtman, 1985). Lewis Thomas has called Alzheimer's disease "the disease of the century" (Thomas, 1981).

THE GREAT INTEREST IN ALZHEIMER'S DISEASE

There are many aspects to Alzheimer's disease that contribute to the extraordinary scientific and public interest it has generated. The by-products alone of Alzheimer's disease research have been very important. Through the new wave of brain studies it has stirred in the search for its cause, a multitude of dramatic new findings about the workings of the brain in general are emerging. It has been a catalyst in the burgeoning new frontier of neuroscience research and in the development of innovative technologies to probe the intricacies of the brain like no other disorder before it. It is contributing essential new pieces to the puzzle of how the brain works and how it becomes dysfunctional.

To behavioral scientists, Alzheimer's disease is being looked at as a new paradigm for studies on the relationships between brain and behavior. One of the remarkable aspects of Alzheimer's disease is that while it represents the unfolding of devastating pathological events in the brain, its major clinical signs and symptoms are behavioral well into the course of the disorder. Unlike other brain diseases such as strokes where you can see physical signs of nerve, motor, and muscular impairment, the external physical appearance of the patient with Alzheimer's disease can look normal for a long time. Instead, the disturbing problems that determine how well and how long one can live in the community or with one's family are cognitive, behavioral, and psychological. They are cognitive in terms of memory and intellectual impairment, behavioral in terms of wandering and agitation, and psychological in terms of depression and delusions. Of historical note, the patient who led Alois Alzheimer to write his classic paper on the disorder in 1906 sought help because of symptoms of paranoid delusions (Alzheimer, 1907). Indeed the absence of apparent physical findings in the early stages of the disorder contributes greatly to the difficulty of diagnosis as well as to the degree of misdiagnosis.

The disorder got its name in 1906 when a German physician named Alzheimer published a paper about this disease. But it was not until some seven decades later that scientific curiosity and public concern about Alzheimer's disease caught fire. Around that time two key changes were occurring. In the public sphere there was developing a fundamental sense of social responsibility to do something about problems of the aging. In the scientific arena the mid-1970s were witnessing a new understanding and interest in separating diseases of later life from changes that represented normal concomitants of the aging process. As part of this latter movement the term "senility," which implied to many an inevitable consequence of growing old, began to give way to terms like senile dementia and Alzheimer's disease, which fostered thinking in the direction of an illness with a cause separate from aging. A whole new set of hypotheses about the etiology of the disorder emerged and hope sprung in the hearts of stricken families of Alzheimer patients. A nation-wide citizens' group was developing in the late 1970s, that became known as the Alzheimer's Disease and Related Disorders Association, and has played a major role since then in keeping national consciousness about this disorder high.

DEFINITION OF THE DISORDER

Alzheimer's disease is a degenerative brain disorder characterized by *dementia*—impairment of memory and other intellectual functions—along with behavioral changes that result from and accompany these deficits. The cause of Alzheimer's disease is unknown. The disorder has a gradual onset and a progressive, deteriorating course, with considerable individual variation as to duration. Corresponding to this clinical picture of the disease are characteristic neuropathological changes identified by microscopic examination of brain tissue; described in Alzheimer's original paper, these changes include neurofibrillary tangles, neuritic plaques, and granulovacuolar degeneration of neurons. Because there are no signs, symptoms, or laboratory findings that are unique to the disorder, apart from the brain tissue (pathological) findings usually not obtained until autopsy, its clinical (as opposed to pathological) diagnosis can be very difficult to make. Many other disorders, ranging from depression to drug side effects, can mimic the clinical manifestations of Alzheimer's disease. Accordingly, the clinical diagnosis of Alzheimer's disease is one of exclusion, where all other specific causes of dementia or dementia-like symptoms must first be ruled out.

Most cases of Alzheimer's disease occur after age 65, striking approximately 6% of this age group in the United States. Hence, it is largely a disease of the aging brain. For reasons that are not clear, Alzheimer's disease appears to be more common in women than in men; this may not entirely be explained by the greater number and increased longevity of older women (women outnumber men 2:1 by age 85). A familial pattern has been described by various investigators, suggesting that heredity may be of some importance; in a small group of families, a genetic linkage marker (see later discussion on genetics, this chapter) has been identified on chromosome 21 of Alzheimer patients. Other researchers emphasize how rudimentary our understanding is of genetic aspects of the disorder. Available data indicate that the likelihood of a close relative developing Alzheimer's disease is four times greater than that in the general population, where the risk is well below 1%. Of course, many disorders have a genetic potential that is either never expressed, partially expressed, or only expressed in combination with other risk factors. There have also been a few reports of a possible association between serious head injuries and the later onset of Alzheimer's disease, though these results are equivocal (Mortimer, French, Hutton, & Schuman, 1985). To date, no other risk factors have been unequivocally identified for Alzheimer's disease.

Alzheimer's disease and related disorders are regarded as being responsible for at least half of the admissions to nursing homes in the United States, with an estimated yearly cost in 1985 dollars in excess of $14 billion for institutional care alone (U.S.D.H.H.S., 1980). Estimates of total direct costs (community home care plus nursing home care) combined with indirect costs (premature death and loss of productivity) come to approximately $88 billion (Huang, Cartwright, & Hu, 1988). Because Alzheimer's disease may so radically alter longevity, many have regarded the disorder as the fourth or fifth leading cause of death (Katzman, Terry, & Bick, 1978).

THEORIES OF CAUSE

Certain mysteries are marked by a multitude of findings that surround them—some of which might take the investigator down the wrong road. Hence, research needs to pay as much attention to identifying which theories will dead end as to which directions will prove promising. The mystery around Alzheimer's disease seems to be accumulating a myriad of clues which hopefully will come together to form a clear picture of what is causing the disorder and what can be done about it. Presently, we are dealing primarily with the hypotheses generated by these clues. The hypotheses essentially fall into five categories, along with a sixth which has been largely dismissed:

1. Unconventional transmissible agent or slow virus theory
2. Vascular theories
3. Chemical and toxin theories
   (a) Chemical deficiencies (e.g., acetylcholine)
   (b) Chemical excesses (e.g., aluminum)
4. Autoimmune theory
5. Genetic theories
6. The largely dismissed theory

Unconventional Transmissible Agent or Slow Virus Theory

Kuru. The search around the globe began with a review of how the cause of a disorder with some clinical and neuropathological similarities to Alzheimer's disease was identified. In the 1950s news of a unique human degenerative brain disease was coming out of New Guinea (Johnson, 1982). A research team, headed by D. Carleton Gajdusek, journeyed out there. Among the striking features of the disorder was its endemic quality, where it was localized almost entirely in a remote tribe of people in the mountains of eastern New Guinea, in the Fore district; a small number of cases were also found in neighboring tribal groups where there had been some intermarriage with the Fore. It was in this area that Melanesian natives were just evolving from a Stone Age mode of existence. The Fore population still lived in barricaded villages, practicing witchcraft and ritualistic cannibalism. The disorder that a growing number of the Fore manifested was known as kuru, which meant "trembling" in the Fore language. It was characterized by progressive ataxia, involuntary movements, muscle weakness and wasting, dementia, and eventually death. No recoveries or remissions have ever been documented.

Initially infection was suspected. But with fever, signs of tissue inflammation, and laboratory findings all absent, consideration was given to other causes—particularly to toxic factors, dietary deficiency, hypersensitivity reactions, autoimmunity, and a purely genetic hypothesis (Gibbs & Gajdusek, 1978). Early suspicion was also directed to the cannibalism as a source of infection, though attention to it diminished when the hypothesis of an infectious origin was dropped. Gajdusek did hold out some question of a pathological process related to hypersensitivity reactions to cannibalized tissues.

Then in 1965, in his laboratory at the National Institutes of Health, Gajdusek discovered that chimpanzees that had been innoculated with tissues from kuru patients developed the same clinical and neuropathological pictures as the afflicted humans—following a delayed onset. Meanwhile, Gajdusek's earlier suspicions about the possible role of hypersensitivity reactions had led Glasse, an anthropologist, to document the very close relationship between the ritualistic practice of cannibalism and the distribution of kuru. Bodies of deceased family members were consumed primarily by adult female relatives and rarely by adult males. Children of both sexes joined their mothers in the ritual. This pattern corresponded to the findings that the disease was most common in women, of equal frequency in boys and girls, and least common in men. Moreover, elders reported that kuru had not been a problem in the tribe before the introduction of cannibalism. The connection between cannibalism and kuru had been missed earlier because the period of time that lapsed between the cannibalistic act and the onset of symptoms could be anywhere from 4 to over 20 years.

These findings by Gajdusek and Glasse reopened both the issue of a potential infection and its possible source. It was not that delayed onset infections of the brain were unknown. In 1905 the spirochete organism causing syphilis was discovered. Subsequently the organism was found in the brains of patients suffering from a syndrome known by such different names as "paresis, dementia paralytica, and general paralysis of the insane" (Harrison et al., 1966). Typically, 10 to 20 years could go by before an untreated infection of syphilis would cause central nervous symptoms. But the infectious process of syphilis differed from the pathology of kuru in several fundamental ways. With syphilis there were signs of the infection in multiple parts of the body, and the organism could be observed in the brain. With kuru, the disease seemed confined to the central nervous system, without signs of infection or isolation of an organism. Upon the successful transmission of kuru to chimpanzees in a manner consistent with an infectious process, Gajdusek attempted again to visualize the organism with the electron microscope. Although this proved to be unsuccessful, the agent was determined to be a virus with atypical qualities.

The fact that a dementing brain disease could be caused by an infectious agent that did not trigger the usual brain and body responses to infection fed speculation that Alzheimer's disease might also be the result of an infectious process, despite the absence of signs of infection with this disorder as well.

Following the cessation of cannibalism among the Fore, kuru began to gradually disappear, with the very few new cases attributed essentially to late onset of the earlier infections. This dramatic decline in the development of new cases in the midst of a large number of individuals already infected and clinically afflicted with the disorder illustrated kuru's unusual lack of conventional communicability. Thus kuru became recognized as the first dementia in man demonstrated to be a virus-induced slow infection with an incubation period measured in years and with a progressive accumulative pathology restricted to the central nervous system, leading to death. It changed the way scientists looked at viral processes and certain brain disorders. It led to a "slow virus" hypothesis for Alzheimer's disease. The history of the effort to understand kuru also illustrates the need and advantage of a multidisciplinary approach to unlocking clues about diseases of unknown cause—the involvement of perspectives as varied as anthropology and neuroscience.

Creutzfeldt-Jakob Disease. Subsequent to the findings in the research on kuru another progressive human dementia, known as Creutzfeldt-Jakob Disease (CJD), was found by Gajdusek to be caused by a slow virus infection with unconventional transmission. The disease is rare, with an incidence of approximately one per million a year (Johnson, 1982). CJD most typically begins in the fifth and sixth decades, but occurs in younger people and those over 65 as well. Its course is usually rapid, with over 80% dying within a year of onset, though some patients have lived with the disorder for as long as 8 years. Like kuru, CJD causes other symptoms beyond the memory and intellectual dysfunction, including ataxia and abnormal motor movements. Hence, both differ from Alzheimer's disease in that they are associated with various neurological signs in addition to the memory and behavioral deficits.

The lack of conventional communicability that is one of the characteristics of kuru is also found with CJD. The infectious nature of the disease was identified in a manner similar to that with kuru, where chimpanzees developed the disorder when innoculated with diseased brain tissue from patients who died from CJD. Of note in the search to identify the cause of CJD was the earlier finding of a familial form of the disorder where 10% to 15% of the cases had a strong family history, with a pattern suggestive of a genetic trait. As a result, a genetic explanation as opposed to an infectious process was initially hypothesized. The discovery of a slow virus infection, on the other hand, need not negate the genetic findings. Instead, the two factors could both have a role in the familial subset of CJD patients; these individuals could have a genetic vulnerability to the disorder which is only expressed in the presence of the slow virus. In the quest to uncover the cause of Alzheimer's disease, two among several hypotheses are the viral and genetic views.

While there is no evidence of CJD being transmitted via typical routes, there are reports of unusual transmissions among humans. One such disturbing report described a recipient of a transplanted cornea developing rapidly progressive CJD 18 months after receiving the transplant from a donor who had died with an undiagnosed brain disorder; subsequent study of the donor's brain revealed CJD (Duffy et al., 1974). This relates to the mode of transmission effected in the laboratory involving innoculations to animals from infected human tissues. Based on these reports of atypical transmissions, warnings have been disseminated about the risk of using corneas or other organs from donors who had an undiagnosed brain disease that might have been of slow virus origin. In recognition of his important pioneering work in demonstrating that kuru and CJD are largely infectious in origin and that the infections are due to the newly regarded slow virus infectious agents, Gajdusek received the Nobel Prize in physiology and medicine in 1976.

Despite clinical similarities observed in comparing Alzheimer's disease with kuru and CJD, neither a slow virus nor any examples of transmission, typical or atypical, have been unequivocally found in cases of Alzheimer victims. Nonetheless, this search has continued, especially within the brain.

Efforts to Observe a Virus. Despite more than 20 years having passed since an infectious origin of kuru was identified, with the findings on CJD following not long thereafter, the slow viral agents in these disorders have yet to be clearly viewed by electron microscopy. Those who hypothesize a slow viral cause for Alzheimer's disease feel that if they can visually identify the slow viruses of kuru and CJD, then they would know better what to look for in attempting to discern a slow virus in electron micrographs of Alzheimer brain tissue. Others have wondered whether, if the virus could not be seen, might not some other structural changes suggestive of the presence of a virus be detected—footprints of the agent, so to speak.

In addition to the two slow virus disorders identified in humans, a third is observed in animals, namely, scrapie in sheep and goats. Electron micrographs of specially stained brain tissues from scrapie infected animals had revealed distinctive particulate structures referred to as *scrapie-associated fibrils* (SAF). A year later, in 1984, a report came out comparing electron micrographs of brain tissues prepared with the same staining technique taken from monkeys infected with scrapie, monkeys infected with kuru, human brain extracts from deceased CJD patients, and human brain extracts from deceased Alzheimer's disease patients. Human brain extracts were taken from patients who had died with other diseases as well to serve as additional controls; these other diseases included parkinsonism dementia, amyotrophic lateral sclerosis (ALS) with dementia, schizophrenia, and cancer. The results were that SAF were observed exclusively in the scrapie, kuru, and CJD tissues—the diseases known to be infected by slow viruses. SAF were not found in the tissues from the patients with Alzheimer's disease or the other disorders. The conclusion of the study was that SAF represented either the etiological agent, a component of the agent, or a product of the pathological processes of the three slow virus diseases. If SAF proved to be the causative agent, the researchers suggested it would represent a new class of filamentous animal virus (Merz et al., 1984). The results also represented another negative finding in the attempt to implicate a slow virus as the cause of Alzheimer's disease, but they have not closed this line of investigation.

Is it a Virus or Other Unconventional Transmissible Agent? Another investigator has questioned whether the infectious agents in scrapie, kuru, and CJD are viruses at all (Prusiner et al., 1983). Prusiner, in raising this question, has also been trying to visualize the infectious agents or traces of them with electron microscopy, and he has attempted to isolate them as well using sophisticated laboratory techniques. He has accumulated considerable data on the agent in scrapie. Remarkable about his findings is that the macromolecule he believes to be the pathogen appears to be a protein entity (referred to as a prion)—not a virus—and not to contain DNA or RNA which all other infectious agents to date are known to possess. If this finding holds up, it would turn upside down some of our most fundamental concepts about infection; prions would represent "a unique and novel class of infectious pathogens." How have prions been looked at in relation to scrapie-associated fibrils (SAF)? It has been suggested that the particulate nature of SAF could represent aggregates of prions (Wurtman, 1985). Prusiner has felt that if the protein he has identified is in fact the scrapie agent, then chemical probes in the form of antibodies to it could be produced. These probes could, in turn, then be used to search for prions in the brains of patients with Alzheimer's disease.

More recently, Prusiner and other investigators have succeeded in developing chemical probes to identify prions in scrapie (Chesebro et al., 1985; Oesch et al., 1985). Moreover, they have found that the protein in prions appears to be found in normal brains as well. This has led to speculation

that prions may function as secondary agents in the infectious process—
not as the primary invaders of the body or brain in the conventional infectious manner. The protein fragment that has been identified in normal
brain tissue may be recruited by an invading virus (e.g., as a protective
capsule for the virus) with the prion being formed in the process and in
turn inducing the pathological changes seen in scrapie. Whether similar
probes will locate any prions in the brains of those with Alzheimer's disease remains to be seen.

That scrapie, kuru, and CJD are all caused by a transmissible agent has
been replicated numerous times. Not resolved is whether the agent is an
atypical virus or some other unconventional agent. Hence, the theory of
an infectious pathogen causing Alzheimer's disease has come to be known
as the unconventional transmissible agent hypothesis.

Still, the unequivocal transmission of Alzheimer's disease to laboratory
animals has not been successful, whether the agent is a slow virus, a
prion, or another unconventional entity.

Other findings continue to keep the transmissible agent hypothesis on a
front burner. A report by Manuelidis et al. (1988) described provocative
results in an experiment where blood from 11 relatives of Alzheimer patients, including two with early signs of Alzheimer's disease, was innoculated intracerebrally into hamsters. The authors reported that in these pilot
experiments, 5 individuals produced brain tissue changes in recipient
hamsters that were similar to pathological changes observed in hamsters
with experimentally induced Creutzfeldt-Jakob disease. The authors, however, emphasized the preliminary nature of the results and that the experiment lacked adequate control comparisons involving healthy age-matched
human subjects without a family history of Alzheimer's disease. In other
words, one cannot tell from this experiment what effect blood from normal
control subjects would have on hamsters—whether human blood in
general injected into hamsters intracerebrally might lead to similar brain
tissue pathology, independent of Alzheimer's disease. There is also the
question of whether human blood causing specific pathological changes in
a different species would cause the same *or any* pathology in other humans.
And, there is the question of whether there was contamination by the CJD
virus in this laboratory where CJD research is also conducted; note that the
brain pathology in these hamsters was that of CJD. Plans for further research involving controls and efforts to see whether the above results could
be replicated were proposed.

Meanwhile, the lesson from the subset of Creutzfeldt-Jakob disease
patients with a familial form of the disorder should not be overlooked. It
was suggested that certain patients with CJD are genetically susceptible
to the disorder if infected with the transmissible agent. It has similarly
been hypothesized that a combination of factors interacting with one

another could be operating in the case of Alzheimer's disease—a transmissible agent being one of the implicated candidates. We are reminded here as well of the contributions of research on the aging brain and its diseases bringing us into contact with dramatic new ideas about the nature of health and illness in general—in this case, the nature of infectious processes and infectious agents. Regardless of the outcome, science is benefiting.

Vascular Theories

One of the earliest contemporary theories of what caused Alzheimer's disease was hardening of the arteries of the brain, or cerebral arteriosclerosis. According to this theory, adequate blood flow to the brain was diminished, resulting in insufficient supply of oxygen to brain tissue. Cognitive impairment was seen as the consequence. Interestingly, many of the present day theories of Alzheimer's disease have historic antecedents in hypotheses of dementia and mental disorder from the distant past. This is particularly relevant to the vascular theory, where at the end of the 18th century the leading explanation of impaired mental functioning was that blood in the brain was sludging. To test this hypothesis an experimental treatment was developed, utilizing a "high tech" apparatus of the late 1700s, known as the "rotating chair" as shown in Figure 6.1. The patient was placed in this special chair which was then rotated at a significant speed in an attempt to relieve the supposed sludging. Unfortunately, this innovation met with a lack of success.

More than a century and a half later, in the late 1960s, a counterpart 20th century high tech apparatus was tested along a related line of reasoning. To improve oxygenation and memory functioning presumably impaired by hardened brain blood vessels, the patient was placed inside the formidable hyperbaric oxygen chamber with oxygen being applied under elevated atmospheric pressure. But here, too, success was not to be achieved. Nonetheless, it was as important to learn what did not work as what did. Families would travel great distances, at great expense, with great hope, only to end up with equally great disappointment and hardship over an ineffective treatment modality. The historical comparison between two conceptually related high tech approaches spanning more than 150 years was also meant to provide an important frame of reference within which to maintain a balanced outlook on the present burgeoning high tech revolution.

Gradually it became recognized that hardening of the arteries did not cause Alzheimer's disease, nor in itself dementia (Clayton & Martin, 1981). Aged individuals could develop significant cerebral arteriosclerosis and maintain good intellectual functioning, or they could have minimal

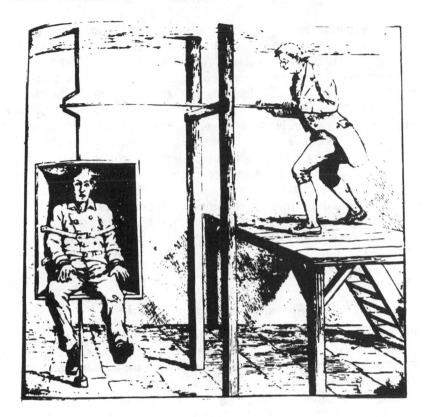

Figure 6.1 The rotating chair circa 1800

arterial impairment and yet reveal advancing Alzheimer's disease. It was not the narrowing of brain blood vessels that resulted in cognitive impairment, but rather the complete blockage that led to a stroke. Hence, attention to vascular factors in dementia shifted from a focus on Alzheimer's disease to one on multiinfarct dementia, a condition of repeated strokes of differing magnitude, at times subtle. Moreover, the vascular pathology leading to multiinfarct dementia was commonly found *outside* the brain, such as in the case of valvular or other heart disease which could cause clot formations that if dislodged could travel to smaller blood vessels in the brain, plugging them up, thereby resulting in a stroke. Hypertension was another risk factor in multiinfarct dementia. While multiinfarct dementia can mimic Alzheimer's disease, it typically has other physical and laboratory findings that can distinguish it.

Though cerebral arteriosclerosis has been dismissed as a possible cause of Alzheimer's disease, other vascular events are being examined. One of

...ways in which the brain is partially protected from various toxins, side effects of certain drugs, and potentially harmful substances in the blood stream is by the so-called *blood-brain barrier,* an anatomically tight junction of membranes between the cells that line the blood vessels and the ventricles of the brain. If blood vessel walls or the blood-brain barrier itself were altered by some pathological process, then the brain could become vulnerable to a range of assaults—viral, toxic, or even immunologic (Fillit, Kemeny, Luine, et al., 1987; Mooradian, 1988; Wisniewski & Merz, 1983). Pathological accumulations of a protein-rich substance known as amyloid have been found in the walls of brain blood vessels in those with Alzheimer's disease, and have been hypothesized as contributing to the pathological events of the disorder (Wurtman, 1985). Meanwhile, the growth of PET scan studies in Alzheimer's disease will likely add a whole new body of information about vascular as well as other ongoing physiologic phenomena associated with the disorder (Frackowiak & Gibbs, 1983).

Chemical and Toxin Theories

With the 20th century has come a resurgence of scientific curiosity about the influence of chemistry on function, rivaling the interest in the study of bodily humors or bodily fluids that captured the clinical imaginations of scientists and clinicians around 500 B.C. These humors were described as being found in the heart, liver, spleen, and brain. An imbalance among them was considered to be the basic cause of disease, and drugs were sought to restore them to their proper proportions (Alexander & Selesnic, 1966). The counterpart to considerations of an imbalance of naturally occurring humors in the brain causing illness in the time of Hippocrates are current concepts of altered levels of neurotransmitters in the brain resulting in the symptoms of Alzheimer's disease.

The Cholinergic Connection: Acetylcholine (ACh). What many scientists consider the most significant clue as to the nature of the underlying problem in Alzheimer's disease was uncovered in the mid-1970s. In 1974 a series of experiments was carried out with healthy young adults to evaluate patterns of memory performance. Some of the experiments used drugs that acted on the brain's cholinergic system, the chemical pathway that produces the neurotransmitter acetylcholine (ACh) (Drachman & Leavitt, 1974). The results were startling. Those drugs that interfered with ACh levels in the brain created temporary memory and behavioral impairments in the young subjects that mimicked those seen in older patients with Alzheimer's disease. When interference with the cholinergic system was stopped, memory functioning returned to normal.

Observations were then made that other drugs also had the side effects of transient intellectual disturbances. The common denominator among these drugs was their potential to lower the level of acetylcholine in the brain. Discontinuing these drugs or counteracting them with other medications resulted in the restoration of baseline performance, presumably as the level of ACh returned to normal. The logical question that followed was that if these experimentally induced conditions of diminished levels of ACh produced a clinical picture resembling Alzheimer's disease in the laboratory, could the basic defect in the actual disorder in nature be one of an ACh deficit?

The answer came in 1976, from two laboratories in the United Kingdom (Davies, 1983). Researchers found that in the cerebral cortex and the hippocampus (the parts of the brain involved with higher intellectual and memory functioning) the level of the enzyme choline acetyltransferase (ChAT) was reduced by as much as 90%. This enzyme being essential for the synthesis of ACh further implicated a deficiency of the neurotransmitter as the key problem in the disease process. Subsequent studies did indeed find marked decrements in the amounts of acetylcholine in the brains of those with Alzheimer's disease as compared to healthy older adults.

Just as the findings of drugs diminishing ACh levels led to the search for a reduction of the neurotransmitter in the disease state, these findings coupled with those of the investigators who discovered ChAT deficits triggered the growth of drug studies aimed at elevating the level of ACh in Alzheimer patients. If drugs could lower the level of ACh and cause memory impairment, could other drugs elevate the level of the neurotransmitter and thereby improve memory functioning in the case of Alzheimer's disease? Parkinson's disease was looked at as a potential model for this approach, in that the various motor symptoms of this disorder were attributed to a deficit in dopamine, another of the brain's neurotransmitters; pharmacologic treatment of parkinsonism with drugs that raise the level of dopamine has resulted in reduced symptomatology.

Choline, Lecithin, Physostigmine, THA. A variety of drugs have been used in an effort to raise ACh levels in patients with Alzheimer's disease. These drugs vary considerably on their mechanisms of action. Choline, lecithin, and physostigmine and THA are among the drugs used that can directly influence the metabolism of ACh. Other drugs act upon the receptor sites which receive the ACh molecules, making these sites more sensitive to the neurotransmitter, and as a result requiring smaller amounts to achieve the same effect. These drugs are being tested alone and in combination with one another. The best result to date with this group of drugs has been with physostigmine taken by itself and in combination with lecithin (Rosenberg, Greenwald, & Davis, 1983) and with

THA (Summers et al., 1986). There have been reports of a small degree of time limited improvement in a limited number of subjects being treated with these drugs; there has not, however, been a significant sustained clinical improvement in these patients to date.

These studies are still in progress. At the same time, research on numerous other pharmacologic agents and somatic interventions are being investigated (Funkenstein et al., 1981). It is important to put these drug studies and experimental procedures into proper perspective.

The public is often puzzled by periodic reports in the press about excitement over new drug trials for Alzheimer's disease, only to be later disappointed in learning that no significant clinical improvement occurs. How then does one explain the excitement? In a number of these instances such enthusiasm has been legitimate, but the nature of the enthusiasm has been misunderstood. If a drug is at all helpful, no matter how small or brief the improvement, it is exciting to the *research* community. To researchers this clinical change suggests that one is potentially on a productive path, one that may lead to a more clinically effective drug, perhaps related to or derivative of the drug being studied (not necessarily the drug being studied). Since the effects at present, however, are not that clinically significant for the family or the physician, there is little excitement in the *practice* community. Such excitement can be legitimate, but one must understand its context and locus, its limitation to the research community for now.

Moreover, it is important not to jump the gun and elevate a theory to a conclusion, or a preliminary finding to a final result, when the facts do not support it. This becomes all the more important when some of the substances being investigated can be purchased over the counter. Often the story behind a new development is much more complicated than the simplified information that first hits the streets. Choline and lecithin are cases in point. Not only have the trials with choline been disappointing, but as dosages were increased, reports emerged of the patients beginning to smell like fish. Lecithin is present in many foods, such as egg yolks, meat, fish, and even certain junk foods. Lecithin sold over the counter, however, is typically quite impure in form, very inadequate in terms of laboratory standards for testing it in Alzheimer patients. Nonetheless, various overzealous commercial enterprizes have advertized it as "food for thought." As awareness and concern about Alzheimer's disease grow, one must be ever cautious about acting too soon on incomplete information when it comes to ingestible substances.

The Nucleus Basalis of Meynert. The cholinergic connection in Alzheimer's disease gathered further strength in 1981 with exciting reports that identified a particular part of the brain known as the nucleus

basalis of Meynert as being specifically affected in the disorder. When the nucleus basalis was studied further its damaged cells were found to be significantly active in the production of acetylcholine (Whitehouse et al., 1981). This provided another piece to the puzzle of Alzheimer's disease, since a circumscribed anatomical change could then be correlated with a key chemical finding in the disorder. In addition, it appeared that there were connecting pathways from the nucleus basalis to the cortical areas of the brain where the classical (described by Alzheimer) neuropathological findings of plaques and tangles were first identified.

It seemed to investigators that the acetylcholine producing nerve cells of the nucleus basalis were very long neurons, with their cell bodies located within the nucleus basalis and their nerve terminals that released the neurotransmitter extending to the cerebral cortex and hippocampus of the brain. It was hypothesized that damage to the nucleus basalis and its cholinergic neurons resulted in ACh deficits within cortical and hippocampal tissues, causing a pathologic process that produced plaque and tangle formations. But what caused damage to the nucleus basalis? Could it be a virus, a toxin, an auto-immune phenomenon, a genetically related event?

Another important aspect about the nucleus basalis finding was that it introduced a fundamentally new way in which Alzheimer's disease was being viewed. Up until that discovery, Alzheimer's disease had generally been regarded as a cortical disorder of the brain. But the nucleus basalis is a subcortical structure, deep within the brain, which accordingly shifted the whole focus in the search for other clues to this mysterious disease process. The finding of a circumscribed lesion also fueled speculation about the potential future application of brain grafts for Alzheimer's disease, following groundbreaking developments with brain tissue transplants to laboratory animals with Parkinson's disease—another brain disease with a specifically affected anatomical site linked to a neurotransmitter deficit. The pathology of Alzheimer's disease, however, appears to be departing from that of Parkinson's disease, in that suspicion is being assigned to additional parts of the Alzheimer brain as having specific anatomical defects or neurochemical deficits. This significantly complicates brain graft considerations.

Other Neurochemical Deficits. Further findings and questions continue to emerge about the involvement in Alzheimer's disease of other neurotransmitters and brain chemicals (Whitehouse, 1987; Perry & Perry, 1985). Two other neurotransmitter deficits in particular have been identified—those of norepinephrine and serotonin—each being linked to pathology at a corresponding anatomical site in the brain. Degenerative changes among Alzheimer patients have been discovered in the *locus coeruleus,* a subcortical nucleus of the brain that is rich in norepinephrine producing neurons. Other pathological changes have been identified in the *dorsal raphé nucleus,* another of the brain's subcortical nuclei, dense in neurons producing serotonin. Like the subcortical nucleus basalis, these subcortical neclei also have neurons whose terminal processes extend to the cerebral cortex.

Of note, too, concerning norepinephrine and serotonin is that these neurotransmitters are also known as biogenic amines, brain chemicals that have been shown to influence emotional states. Since depression and delusions are commonly described in different Alzheimer patients, attention to these other neurotransmitter changes becomes all the more important in understanding what might be contributing to the behavioral problems of the disorder and what approaches might be taken to alleviate them.

In Chapter 8, there is a substantial discussion of the different neurochemical and neuroanatomical events that take place with neurons that appear to have a major role in brain plasticity. Particularly emphasized are substances such as *nerve growth factors,* chemical compounds that have *neurotrophic* functions—that is, they have the ability to influence the metabolic activities of nerve cells. Various investigators have wondered whether if the application of neurotrophic agents had a positive effect on brain plasticity, could a deficit in one or more of these agents have a deleterious effect and be playing a role in Alzheimer's disease (Kosei & Appel, 1983). Here, too, identification of a specific neurotrophic chemical deficiency would have ramifications for potential pharmacologic replacement interventions.

Another neurochemical, *somatostatin,* classified as a neuropeptide, has been found to be diminished in different parts of the brain of Alzheimer victims. Two other aspects of somatostatin have taken on added interest in light of the above discussion. First, among the different sites in the brain where somatostatin has been located is the nucleus basalis. This has led some researchers to question whether somatostatin might play a part in effecting the changes seen with Alzheimer's disease in the basal nucleus. Second, a possible role of somatostatin in influencing neurotrophic factors has also been raised, tying in with inquiries about neurotrophic deficits in the disorder.

Aluminum. Moving from theories that examine chemical deficiencies to explain the cause of Alzheimer's disease, we come to others that are looking at toxic excesses of various substances. Aluminum has commanded the most visibility in this area (Perl, 1983). A number of studies have identified an increased amount of aluminum in the brains of those with Alzheimer's disease. Given that aluminum is the most abundant metallic element in our environment has added to the concern as to whether or not it plays a part in the genesis of the disorder. With many of the changes that are observed in Alzheimer's disease, and in the case of aluminum in particular, there is a critical question that must immediately be raised: Is the change a cause or an effect of the disorder? Is the accumulation of aluminum in Alzheimer brains an indication of a toxic impact of the metal, or is its buildup simply a consequence of pathologic changes in the diseased tissue that allow aluminum to incidentally accrue? Increasingly the latter appears to be the case—that increased aluminum in Alzheimer's disease is an effect, not a cause, of the disorder (Terry, 1985; Wurtman, 1985).

The search for additional evidence about the role of aluminum has not only taken investigators into the brain, but into the neuron itself where aluminum has been found in conjunction with the classic neurofibrillary tangles of the disorder. The healthy neuron contains within its axon and dendrites smaller fibrils with a protein composition (see Figure 2.3). There are different subgroups of these neurofibrils, each with certain characteristic features as to shape and diameter. The neurofibrillary tangles seen in Alzheimer's disease are also located within the neuron, but here the tangles clearly assume a different form from the normal neurofibrils, a configuration of *paired helical filaments* (PHFs). As implied by their name, these PHFs consist of pairs of neurofibrils spirally twisted into a helical pattern; they are also of a different diameter than normal neurofibrils. Hence, the form and diameter of the tangles allow them to be readily distinguished from normal neuronal structures under the electron microscope. Evidence is mounting that the protein composition of the PHFs differs from normal neurofibrils, the former appearing "to be derived from a complex alteration of normal cytoskeletal elements" of the latter (Selkoe, 1986, p. 429).

Did aluminum wreak havoc on the neurofibrils within the neuron, causing them to tangle, or did the tangles exert an affinity for aluminum which attracted the element into the diseased nerve cell? Part of the detective work to resolve this "which came first" dilemma involved studying the effects of aluminum on the brain cells of laboratory animals. Aluminum injections were administered to the brains of cats and rabbits. Interestingly, tangles did form. But they differed anatomically from the PHFs seen in Alzheimer's disease in four important ways. The experimentally induced tangles had only one strand, as opposed to a pair; they were not helical in shape; they had a different diameter than the PHFs; and they were found in parts of the brain not affected in Alzheimer's disease (Reisberg, 1981).

Further human evidence serving to *not* implicate aluminum in Alzheimer's disease comes from renal dialysis studies. Patients on chronic renal dialysis are at risk of developing a dialysis dementia which actually is attributed to the aluminum in the dialysate solution. The pathological brain changes that result, however, do not correspond to those of Alzheimer's disease, nor does the clinical picture. Despite the presence of brain concentrations of aluminum being higher in the dialysis dementia, no plaques and tangles are caused by this elevation. The suspicion of aluminum as the culprit in Alzheimer's disease does not hold up under the weight of these findings—certainly not as an agent acting alone.

Yet more evidence weighing against aluminum has come forth from around the continent. Early reports about elevated aluminum concentrations in the brain of Alzheimer patients originated from studies in Toronto, Canada and in Burlington, Vermont. Subsequently, cases of Alzheimer's disease from Lexington, Kentucky showed normal concentrations of aluminum, but the Kentucky report also pointed out that the other two geographic regions had high concentrations of aluminum in their drinking water due to the use of alum for purification purposes— a practice not followed in Lexington, Kentucky. From these findings it has been inferred that aluminum excess in some tissue specimens from Alzheimer victims could be an epiphenomenon rather than a causal one (Terry, 1985). It should also be pointed out that numerous studies of aluminum have failed to uncover toxic effects in general; unusual circumstances, such as with some patients on renal dialysis, represent the only exceptions. Similarly, as far as the use of aluminum pots and pans is concerned, studies show very little interaction between food and aluminum utensils, which continue to appear to be very safe indeed (Sorenson et al., 1974). Still, the idea of aluminum having some role in Alzheimer's disease has not been put entirely to rest by some investigators.

A68: A Protein More Common in Alzheimer Brains? One of the most intriguing recent findings has been that of a protein, differing from a prion, initially identified to be in significantly greater quantities in the brains of those with Alzheimer's disease as compared to normals (Wolozin, Pruchnicki, Dickson, & Davies, 1986; Barnes, 1987). The protein, referred to as A68, may provide fascinating new clues. Further analysis of A68 could offer new insights into the cause of Alzheimer's disease, and possibly lead to an important new diagnostic test for the disorder. Researchers might, for example, be able to determine whether A68 comes from a virus, whether it represents a protein of the normal brain transformed by autoimmune or toxic factors, or whether some other pathologic process induces its formation.

Moreover, A68 has also been identified in cerebrospinal fluid (CSF). If the finding of its relative uniqueness holds up, it could eventually result in the first specific practical diagnostic test for Alzheimer's through clinical evaluation of CSF. In general, its discovery re, one of the latest new impetuses in the vigorous search for cause.

Autoimmune Theory

The exploration for autoimmune phenomena has become pronounced in the 20th century, though the concept is not new, especially with regard to the brain. Emil Kraepelin, one of the 19th century pioneers in the history of psychiatry and neurology, postulated that brain injury could be caused by an unknown metabolite which he called an "auto-toxin" (Alexander & Selesnic, 1966). Current concepts of autoimmunity look at the individual's immune system as somehow becoming fooled into thinking that part of one's own body is a foreign agent, like a bacterial infection, and attacking it. Consideration of an autoimmune phenomenon to explain the onset of Alzheimer's disease has led to the search for antibrain antibodies in these patients.

It has been speculated that due to the progressive aging of brain neurons, which do not replicate after early childhood, late life changes in these cells may fool the organism's immune system into thinking that foreign bodies are present. An autoimmune response might then be triggered. In fact, antibodies against brain tissue have been found in the blood streams of those with Alzheimer's disease. But such antibodies are observed in the bloodstreams of normal older adults as well (Lauter, 1985). To a large extent they are believed to be kept from having direct contact with brain tissue by the blood-brain barrier. Of course, if the integrity of the blood-brain barrier were altered, this equilibrium could be upset. This point was alluded to earlier in the discussion of vascular hypotheses as to the genesis of Alzheimer's disease.

Immunological considerations in Alzheimer's disease have also focused closely on another of the classic neuropathological findings of the disorder—the *plaques,* also known as senile plaques, neuritic plaques, or amyloid plaques. Investigators report that the concentration of plaques in the brain closely correlates with the degree of dementia exhibited by Alzheimer patients. Plaques consist of three components: parts (debris) from degenerating neurons, nonneuronal (scavenger) cells of the brain that react to this degenerative process, and amyloid (Wisniewski, 1983). Literature in general on amyloid suggests that it is deposited under conditions of altered immunity, while immunoglobulins (antibodies, protein in nature) have been identified in the amyloid of the plaques seen in Alzheimer's disease (Lauter, 1985).

Just as the triggering of neurofibrillary tangle formation is not understood, what induces plaques to form similarly remains a mystery. Do plaques and/or tangles represent the work of a virus, or the outcome of an immunologic reaction to a transmissible agent at the cellular level? Do genetic defects that are only expressed with aging result in the formation of abnormal proteins in neurons which in turn trigger an autoimmune response? Other findings suggest that the brain in Alzheimer's disease may be deficient in RNA, the nucleic acid found in the nucleus of a neuron that mediates the translation of the genetic code of DNA in manufacturing protein for the nerve cell; could errors result from this defect, with autoimmune consequences? (Sajdel-Sulkowska & Marotta, 1984). But what would have caused the RNA deficiency? The web is truly complicated.

Genetic Theories

Before examining the genetic theories about Alzheimer's disease, some considerations relevant to genetics and illness in general should be briefly reviewed. First, the fact that certain diseases occur more in some families than in others does not necessarily mean the disorder has a genetic basis. As family members live in very close proximity to one another, they could easily be exposed to the same transmissible agent or environmental toxin, which could explain why some families might be more affected than others by various illnesses. Second, a genetic component to an illness does not necessarily mean the disorder is an hereditary illness; it could be congenital—due to a prenatal or developmental physiologic phenomenon, not brought on by heredity. During fetal development, for example, DNA (the coded genetic information controlling cellular events) in brain neurons could be damaged, without comparable changes occurring in the individual's reproductive cells where hereditary phenomena are governed. A tissue specific injury, chemical deficiency, virus, or toxin, for example, could affect the DNA in one set of cells and not another; this would be an acquired (a developmental) as opposed to an inherited genetic defect. Circumstances of this nature were touched upon in the preceding discussion of autoimmune considerations. Third, an individual could have an inherited genetic potential to develop a disorder, but in the absence of other factors acting to trigger the release of this genetic potential, it might never be expressed. Such an interaction of factors is suggested in the case of that subset of patients with Creutzfeldt-Jakob disease who appear to have a genetic tendency for the disorder, which only becomes expressed under the influence of the slow virus infection.

Genetic interest in Alzheimer's disease has been further stirred, however, by an association between the occurrence of this disorder and Down's syndrome among different members of the same family. Though a basic understanding of this association remains elusive, it has led to efforts to identify a genetic marker for Alzheimer's disease on chromosome 21—the

chromosome affected in Down's syndrome. Such efforts have gaine\
tional momentum given the existence of a small group of families wh\
autosomal dominant trait (hereditary expression of one of the ch...omo-
somes not involved in determining the sex of the individual) appears to be
operating (Briley, Chopin, & Moret, 1986). Genetic subtypes now appear
even more likely with the discovery of a genetic linkage marker (common
chromosomal finding in patients with a strong family history of a disorder)
on chromosome 21 in the autosomal dominant families (St George-Hyslop,
Tanzi, Polinski, et al., 1987). But the extent of genetic and hereditary
involvement as a whole in families with Alzheimer's disease remains
unclear because of the vast number affected with the disorder who do not
manifest autosomal dominant disease patterns or clear-cut genetic features (Davies, 1986).

Heston (1983) studied families from the subset of Alzheimer patients in
whom an inherited potential to develop the disorder appeared to exist
(the autosomal dominant group). He found that an apparent genetic
potential does not mean at all that if one family member develops the
disorder, the others will as well. Even when there appears to be some
hereditary history for Alzheimer's in a given family, the likelihood remains relatively low for any specific individual in that family to develop
the disorder. However, though their risk is low, it is greater than with the
general population. In the nonhereditary group, the risk of a relative
developing the disorder is apparently similar to that of the general population. In the hereditary group, if one family member has the disorder the
approximate risk of close relatives (children, siblings, parents) later experiencing or already having developed the illness is 3–6% at ages 65–69, as
compared to 0.5% for the general population in that age range; 11–13%
for relatives aged 75–79, as compared to 2.5% for the general population
in that age range; 19–22% for relatives aged 85–89, as compared to 6.5%
for the general population in that age range. Risks are much lower for
more distant relatives, and the figures are quite small in general for relatives under age 65. Moreover, in families where someone has Alzheimer's
disease, regardless of age at onset, it is reported that if another member of
that family develops the disorder it is likely to occur at a later age for that
individual (Lauter, 1985).

Down's Syndrome. A small but significant increase in the incidence of
Down's syndrome has been found in families with Alzheimer's disease.
Furthermore, studies show that the classic neuropathological changes of
Alzheimer's disease, including plaques and tangles, are found in the
brains of virtually 100% of individuals with Down's over the age of 35.
Curiously, despite this neuropathological correlation, less than a third of
the Down's individuals in this age group manifested the clinical picture

of dementia on top of their basic disorder; the reason for this discrepancy between brain and behavioral manifestations is not understood (Wisniewski et al., 1985). More fundamentally, though, the significance of an association between Alzheimer's disease and Down's syndrome is not understood, except in terms of an hypothesized genetic connection.

Even when one does not know the significance of a new finding, the consideration of it as a potential clue to a greater discovery can bring to the investigator's mind very important questions that might otherwise never have been raised. This is one of the generically most exciting aspects of research in general—the sequence of a curious fragment of information pointing to new directions for study, at times leading to a fundamental breakthrough in the solution of a major problem for mankind. This has also been the pattern of research in the area of Alzheimer's disease, where a myriad of clues are being uncovered. While they have not as yet added up to identify the cause and cure for the disorder, they have provided the researcher with a range of highly relevant new areas for exploration. Aspects of this phenomenon can be found with each of the theories as to the cause of Alzheimer's disease. The relationship between Alzheimer's disease and Down's syndrome also illustrates this point by having raised two very important clinical questions that had not previously been considered. The first focuses on chromosome 21, the second on maternal age.

Because studies of the underlying pathology in Down's syndrome identified the involvement of chromosome 21 at the cellular level as influencing the disease process, and because of the association between Down's syndrome and Alzheimer's disease, investigators have focused in on chromosome 21 in Alzheimer's disease as well. Chromosomes, of course, house genes which in turn consist of various DNA genetic coding sequences. Finding abnormalities in chromosome 21 in Alzheimer's disease could potentially lead to the first specific laboratory test for making a definitive diagnosis of the disorder other than neuropathological study of the brain usually done at autopsy. Since chromosomes are found in all the cells of the body, one would not have to use brain tissue; one could use skin cells, for example, in a straightforward diagnostic procedure with the living patient. If an abnormal sequence of genetic coding were identified on chromosome 21, one could then similarly make the diagnosis prenatally, via amniocentesis, with the obvious ramifications that this approach would create. The initial chromosome 21 findings in Alzheimer's disease require further replication. Of course, even if replicated, they still might be found in only a small subgroup of families with the disorder. Meanwhile, a specific and reliable diagnostic test has not developed from these findings. Nonetheless research interest in this area is very high and growing.

Ultimately, if an abnormal genetic coding sequence in Alzheimer's disease were identified, whether on chromosome 21 or elsewhere, it could eventually lead to progress in interventions along several fronts. The opportunities for developing a specific diagnostic test, genetic counseling, and prenatal intervention have already been alluded to. Conceivably, too, through progress in molecular biology, abnormal genetic coding sequences could in the future be corrected, with the consequent opportunities for both cure and prevention. But first, such abnormal sequences must be found (the genetic linkage marker that has been identified may not be abnormal, but associated with something else unknown that is).

A second major clinical question that arises from the association between Alzheimer's disease and Down's syndrome centers on maternal age. With Down's syndrome, maternal age is a risk factor. The chances of a Down's baby being born increase with the advancing age of the mother at childbirth. Does the same risk hold for Alzheimer's disease? Is there a greater frequency of Alzheimer's disease in those born from older mothers? A carefully controlled study looked at this question, and expanded it by not only examining maternal age, but paternal age as well (Corkin, Growdon, & Rasmussen, 1983). The results indicated that patients with Alzheimer's disease and nondemented control subjects did not differ in the average ages of their parents at the time of the patients' or subjects' births. This applied to mothers and fathers alike. Hence, more advanced maternal or paternal age with the birth of a child was *not* found to increase the risk of that child later developing Alzheimer's disease. Furthermore, no relationship was found between parental age and either early onset (before age 65) or later onset (65 and older) Alzheimer's disease. Other studies have confirmed these findings of no relation between parental age and risk for Alzheimer's disease (White, McGue, & Heston, 1986). The public health ramifications of parental age being a risk factor would have been significant, especially with changing trends of professional women in the work force and later childbearing years.

The latter example points out how it can be as important to rule out something as a risk factor, as it is to rule it in. It was a highly relevant question to have been raised. Also highlighted by the discovery of a relationship between Alzheimer's disease and Down's syndrome is the potential contribution of research on aging to new insights about disorders at other points in the life cycle; it is possible that a breakthrough in the treatment of Alzheimer's disease could also contribute to the treatment of Down's syndrome.

STILL A MYSTERY

Theories of what causes Alzheimer's disease have not been lacking. Clues are myriad and mounting. But the solution as to its etiology is still elusive. It is in the nature of how we look for problems as well as solutions that we seek the starting *point,* the single critical event. In much of life and disease this seemingly reductionistic approach often pays off. A complex human being comes from a single fertilized one-cell ovum. Fever, sweating, headache, cough, respiratory congestion, nasal discharge, muscle and joint aches and pains, rapid pulse beat, rash, swollen glands, weakness, fatigue, nausea, vomiting, diarrhea, trouble sleeping, along with other symptoms all occurring at the same time can be entirely explained by a solitary influenza viral infection.

But sometimes in life and medicine the single causative factor cannot explain everything. The genetic evidence suggests more than one subtype of Alzheimer's disease; the findings from studies of Creutzfeldt-Jakob disease show how two factors (genetics and a virus) can interact to cause a degenerative brain disorder resembling Alzheimer's disease; clinical courses of varying durations among those afflicted with Alzheimer's disease may also suggest the role of multiple factors effecting this variability. With all of this said and summarized, the origin of Alzheimer's disease remains a mystery. But the race to solve it is picking up ever faster, as the pieces to its puzzle continue to increase and to connect. Scientists hope the answers for "the disease of the century" will come before the end of the century.

7

Diagnosis and Treatment of Alzheimer's Disease

Whereas, on the one hand, research on Alzheimer's disease (AD) is expanding our understanding of basic brain processes, on the other hand it is providing new insights into the nature and treatment of behavioral problems. As alluded to in the preceding chapter, AD offers a paradigm for examining relationships between brain phenomena and behavioral manifestations. Important new insights about such relationships are likely to come from the mounting studies in this area. Because so many of the major clinical problems in AD are behavioral in nature for so much of its clinical course, treatment planning and research on AD must pay particular attention to behavioral issues (Teri, Larson, & Reifler, 1988; Merriam, Aronson, Gaston, Wey, & Katz, 1988). It has also been suggested that the clinical problems confronted in treating AD are of such magnitude and complexity that progress here will translate into an improved state of the art for the treatment of chronic illnesses in general, and especially for chronic mental disorders.

A great disservice is done to Alzheimer patients and their families by statements that say there is no treatment for AD or senile dementia. What such comments actually mean is that there is no cure. The proper perspective on treatment for a severe disorder like AD emphasizes the dichotomy between cure and care in conceptualizing an overall plan for intervention. The fact is that there are a host of clinical interventions that can be utilized to treat the patient with this disorder. While it is true that the clinician cannot prevent, reverse, or stop the progression of AD, the ways in which the patient and his or her family live through this progression can be significantly helped through a range of treatment approaches. Symptoms and suffering can be diminished, coping skills assisted, the dignity of the patient and family preserved. These should be goals in any treatment plan. They have been too long overlooked in the case of AD, where there is much opportunity for treatment beyond care alone. Again, this is a concept that applies to a wide range of chronic disorders.

HISTORY

The attempt to develop systematic and aggressive treatment strategies for AD represents a rather recent historical phenomenon. In 1978 three national institutes (The National Institute of Mental Health, The National Institute on Aging, and the National Institute of Neurological and Communicative Disorders and Stroke) co-sponsored a landmark international conference to consolidate what was known and to establish a research agenda for clinical approaches to AD. The findings and recommendations that focused on intervention strategies from that conference were organized into four categories: treatment, management, models of service delivery, and social policy implications (Miller & Cohen, 1981). Treatment approaches were organized into behavioral, environmental, and somatic interventions; service delivery models examined the potential contributions of both formal and informal support systems. These elements offer a useful outline for comprehensive treatment planning broadly.

The determination and vigor generated among researchers and clinicians in the late 1970s were also igniting within families. In 1980, The Alzheimer's Disease and Related Disorders Association (ADRDA) was founded, with a strong focus on and involvement of families. ADRDA is a privately funded national voluntary health organization that has grown to more than 500 support groups and over 125 chapters nationwide (Stone, 1987). Its international counterpart, Alzheimer's Disease International, was established in 1984. The growth of ADRDA has also been accompanied by the development of an important new literature on treatment and care for AD, designed to assist families and geared to a general public readership (Mace & Rabins, 1981; Heston & White, 1983; Cohen & Eisdorfer, 1986).

Why did it take so long for a vigorous approach to better treatment and care for AD to be launched? After all, the disorder had been formally named and described as a disease during the first decade of the century. Part of the problem was that the patient described in Alois Alzheimer's classic case was only 51 years of age. It was not until the 1970s, with the recognition that the pathological brain tissue changes observed in the small number of patients under age 65 with AD were the same as the majority of those with dementia over 65, that the term Alzheimer's disease became widely used with the elderly patients.

Scientific interest then expanded from a fascination with the intriguing plaques and tangles in the brains of AD victims to an awareness of how the disorder's behavioral symptomatology created treatment opportunities for patients and families. All of this coincided with the burgeoning of geriatrics as a new field of medical research and practice in the mid-1970s—a field very much interested in separating changes that represented illness in the older person from those that reflected normal aging. What had previously been passively accepted as the expected senility of growing old, was now being understood as AD, a clinical disorder demanding treatment.

THE APPROACH TO TREATMENT PLANNING

Building upon the elements of a comprehensive treatment plan as introduced above, the following outline could be considered in developing an overall intervention strategy for AD:

1. Establishing the proper diagnosis
2. Contemplating the clinical course
3. Treating the patient's symptoms
4. Intervening with significant others
5. Addressing the patient's environment
6. Reviewing the role of the service system
7. Examining social policy

Establishing the Proper Diagnosis (Differential Diagnosis)

Because there are as yet no clinical tests that specifically indicate the presence of AD, its diagnosis can be very difficult to establish, particularly at its onset. If the diagnosis of AD is suspected, the burden on the clinician is to prove that some other disease whose symptoms closely resemble those of AD is not present; such is the process of making a diagnosis by exclusion.

A multitude of other disorders can masquerade as AD. Since so many clinical problems can mimic Alzheimer's disease, misdiagnosis occurs in both directions—diagnosing AD when the problem is that of another disorder, or diagnosing another illness when it is really AD. It is estimated that as many as 15% to 30% of those who present with dementia-like symptoms are incorrectly diagnosed, especially early in the course of their illnesses (National Institute on Aging Task Force, 1980). Accurate diagnosis is essential, since it affects the choice of treatments as well as expectations and planning for the patient's future. The push for accurate diagnosis has indeed been great with AD, an effort that is paving new pathways in how we examine cognition, ideation, affect, and behavior in attempting to assess brain function (Reisberg, 1983). This push is also serving to sharpen how we look at the borderlands between normal cognition and cognitive impairment in later life. It brings us into contact with descriptions of such later life phenomena as pseudodementia and benign senescent forgetfulness.

Pseudodementias and Conditions That Can Mimic AD. Dementia-like symptoms of altered memory, concentration, and intellectual functioning occur in psychological as well as physical disorders, and consequently can mislead the observer about the true nature of the underlying problem. Various studies have shown, for example, that as many as 15% to 20% of depressed older adults exhibit signs of transient cognitive impairment (Roth, 1978; Caine, 1981); in its severe form, this condition has been referred to as a pseudodementia. Other pseudodementias and conditions that can be misdiagnosed as AD include drug side effects, alcoholism, psychotic states (e.g., late life schizophrenia), metabolic disorders (e.g., thyroid disease), nutritional deficiency states (e.g., thiamine deficiency), covert infections, cardiovascular problems, stroke, head trauma, brain tumors, secondary symptoms from loss of hearing or vision, various other brain disorders, and even complications from social isolation. Many of these masquerading problems can be cured or brought under clinical control.

The Major Categories of Dementia in the Elderly. When the diagnosis of dementia is correct in the elderly, AD is the most common but not the only cause. Approximately 50% of dementias in older adults are caused by AD; approximately 20% are caused by strokes (multi-infarct dementia); approximately 18% are caused by AD and multi-infarct dementia in combination; the rest are caused by a sizeable group of miscellaneous disorders (Wang, 1981; Sloane, 1980). Hence, in about two-thirds of the dementias seen in this age group, AD has a part—and in one-third it does not.

A new source of dementia that will require careful monitoring is that of AIDS (acquired immune deficiency syndrome). While the frequency of AIDS dementia in the elderly is not known, some data on the frequency of AIDS in older adults is available. One study found 10% of AIDS positive cases to be 50 years of age or older, 2.5% of AIDS positive cases to be 60 years of age or older, and 0.4% of AIDS positive cases to be 70 years of age or older; the source of the infection was three times as great from transfusions as from homosexual contact (Moss & Miles, 1987).

Benign Senescent Forgetfulness (Age-Associated Memory Impairment).
The diagnosis of AD is difficult to make not only because one has to rule
out all of the disorders that can mimic its symptoms, but also because of
the need to document pathological decline over time. In this regard there
is a form of mild memory impairment, identified by Kral and seen in a
number of older adults, that is largely indistinguishable from the early
stage of AD. Referred to as "benign senescent forgetfulness" (Kral, 1978)
or as "age-associated memory impairment" (Crook et al., 1986), individuals with this condition experience intermittent difficulty recalling names,
places, dates, and parts of past events; at other times, they do not display
any trouble remembering the same items. At worst, this condition seems to
progress relatively slowly, differing dramatically from the severe deterioration and eventual incapacity of AD.

Transient Cognitive Impairment. Both puzzling and intriguing was
the clinical course of another group of elderly individuals identified in the
Duke Longitudinal Study I of Aging. Intellectual functioning was one of
a number of parameters followed over a 21-year period in this landmark
research effort. Repeated findings were reported on a significant number
of older adults who when tested in one year had documented cognitive
impairment, whereas upon retesting in a subsequent year no longer revealed this impairment (Busse, 1978). Explanations remained elusive.
Here, too, the significance of a period of time having to pass (to document
deterioration) before a diagnosis of AD can be reached at its early stage is
vividly illustrated. What at first looks very much like the gradual onset of
AD, may later turn out not to be the case.

Everyday Forgetfulness in Later Life. Not to be overlooked is the
question of whether, despite complaints, there is really any cognitive
change at all. Around age 50 an interesting phenomenologic event takes
place. Concerns about memory or forgetfulness begin to rise, in part
because of expectation as opposed to actual occurrence of difficulty.
There is an increased tendency to observe oneself in a search for signs of
"senility." If periods of memory trouble do occur, they are often temporary, such as with bereavement or any stressful situation that makes it
hard to concentrate. At other times, older people are often accused or
accuse themselves of memory changes which are not really taking place.
If a person in his thirties misplaces keys or a wallet, forgets the name of a
neighbor, or calls one sibling by another's name, nobody gives it a second
thought. But the same normal forgetfulness in people in their sixth
decade and beyond may raise unjustifiable concern. An interesting finding from research on those who complain excessively about memory
difficulties, in the absence of identifiable intellectual impairment, is that

such individuals may well have an underlying depression (Kahn, Zarit, Hilbert, & Niederehe, 1975; Plotkin, Mintz, & Jarvik, 1985). This differs from pseudodementia where cognitive changes are found. Whereas some people express emotional stress via somatic symptoms, a number of older adults signal inner turmoil through memory complaints.

The Diagnostic Work-Up. Any older person with noticeable memory problems, trouble concentrating, or disturbances in their thinking or intellectual functioning should receive a comprehensive differential diagnostic evaluation. There are three major components to this work-up: general medical, neurological, and psychiatric/neuropsychological. The specific tests and procedures within this broad framework continue to be the subject of intense study and review. For example, in the spring of 1983 a Secretarial Task Force on AD was established by the U.S. Department of Health and Human Services (DHHS), with a report elaborating directions for research and including a section on diagnosis published in 1984 (USDHHS, 1984). Under the auspices of this Task Force, a special multidisciplinary Work Group was also formed to elaborate clinical approaches to the diagnosis of AD. This Work Group attempted to develop clinical criteria for making *possible, probable,* and *definite* diagnoses of AD, with their report also published in 1984 (McKhann et al., 1984). Their table summarizing these clinical criteria is reproduced in the Appendix as Table A-1.

Other researchers/clinicians have also developed general guidelines for carrying out comprehensive diagnostic evaluations of patients suspected of having AD (Gustafson, 1985; Reisberg & Ferris, 1982; Sloane, 1980; Wang, 1981; Wells, 1982). These guidelines have several elements in common. They include a thorough medical history and clinical examination (with attention to general physical, neurological, and psychiatric signs and symptoms); laboratory blood and urine studies (including a complete blood count, a standard metabolic screening battery with serum enzymes and electrolytes, thyroid function studies, vitamin B and folate levels, and a serological test for syphilis); a chest x-ray; and when indicated (if the preceding tests have not established the diagnosis) such special studies as an electroencephalogram (EEG) and a CAT (computerized axial tomography) scan.

Certain other techniques that have received more research than clinical attention in the area of AD are the PET (positron emission tomography) scan and MRI (magnetic resonance imaging, previously referred to as NMR). In 1987, an NIH (National Institutes of Health) Consensus Conference on Dementing Disorders attempted to tackle the problem of what tests should be considered for the differential diagnosis of dementing disorders in the standard evaluation of a patient with symptoms of dementia; the recommendations are included in the Appendix in Table A-2.

Brief screening tests have attracted considerable interest in efforts to diagnose dementia in general and to differentiate between different types of dementia. Commonly used brief mental status questionnaires used to establish a preliminary diagnosis of the presence of dementia or organically caused cognitive impairment include the Mini-Mental State developed by Folstein and colleagues (Folstein, Folstein, & McHugh, 1975), the Short, Portable Mental Status Questionnaire, developed by Pfeiffer (Pfeiffer, 1975), and a 10-question test popularized by Kahn and Goldfarb (Kahn, Goldfarb, Pollack, & Peck, 1960). The latter two are particularly brief and are presented in Tables 7.1 and 7.2. These tests are far from definitive, and are viewed as helpful mainly in raising the *possibility* of dementia like that of AD; once the suspicion of AD or any other dementia is raised, more extensive testing should follow. If a diagnosis of dementia is arrived at, the question arises as to which one. Because after AD the second most common dementia in later life is that of multi-infarct dementia, tests have been sought to distinguish between these two disorders. Hachinski and colleagues developed an "ischemic score" with the goal of differentiating between multi-infarct dementia and AD (Hachinski, 1983); complicating this differentiation has been the finding that approximately as many patients have these two disorders together as those who have multi-infarct dementia alone.

Table 7.1 Mental Status Questionnaire for Cognitive Impairment [a]

1. Where are we now?
2. Where is this place located?
3. What month is it?
4. What day of the month is it?
5. What year is it?
6. How old are you?
7. What is your birthday?
8. Where were you born?
9. Who is the President of the United States?
10. Who was President before him?

[a] Scoring: 0–2 errors suggest no or mild cognitive impairment; 3–8 errors, moderate impairment; 9–10 errors, severe impairment.

Source: Kahn, Goldfarb, Pollack, & Peck (1960). Reproduced by permission.

Table 7.2 Short Portable Mental
Status Questionnaire [a]

1. What is the name of this place?
2. What is your street address? *OR* What is your telephone number?
3. What is the date today?
4. What day of the week is it?
5. How old are you?
6. When were you born?
7. Who is the President of the United States now?
8. Who was the President before him?
9. What was your mother's maiden name?
10. Subtract 3 from 20 and keep subtracting 3 from each new number all the way down.

[a] Scoring: 0–2 errors suggest no or mild cognitive impairment; 3–8 errors, moderate impairment; 9–10 errors, severe impairment.

Source: Pfeiffer (1975). Reproduced by permission.

Contemplating the Clinical Course

Alzheimer's disease presents a major treatment challenge, not just because of the magnitude of symptomatology and dysfunction that accompany it, but also because its clinical course changes over time; this results in varying problems that demand ongoing adjustments in the nature, mix, and timing of interventions. Its natural history, in short, confronts one with both chronicity and flux—ultimate tests for treatment planning. Consequently, treatment plans for AD must address long-term care and progressive clinical course considerations.

An understanding of the clinical course of AD allows patients, families, and service providers the opportunity to plan in advance for interventions that can lessen the burden on all involved. In general, this clinical course is characterized by gradually worsening memory, intellectual functioning, and capacity to carry out activities of everyday living. At the early stage of the illness changes may be unrecognized by most people, though the patient is usually aware of increased forgetfulness and difficulty naming persons and objects; trouble with social and work-oriented activities is generally not apparent. By the final stage, one's reasoning abilities and orientation in the world are drastically deteriorated; incontinence and a total inability to care for oneself ensue.

Early intellectual changes may include difficulties in previously trouble-free areas, such as in balancing the checkbook. Memory problems slowly become more noticeable, often at first to oneself and then to others. As memory deteriorates further, one may forget phone messages, confuse dates, and misplace things. It may get increasingly difficult to find the right word to name or describe something, and one may forget the first chapters in the book one is reading. Typically, recent memory (such as what one had for breakfast) appears more impaired than remote memory (e.g., high school events). Memory impairment can become dangerous, as in forgetting to shut off the gas stove or to lock one's door, or which way to turn at the top of a stairway.

Vague personality or behavior changes may be observed as the disorder slowly begins to progress. The individual may seem to be losing motivation or manifesting a sense of apathy with others, or at other times, restlessness and a reduced attention span might be observed. New, annoying traits might appear, such as suspiciousness or contrariness. Family members, friends, colleagues caught by surprise with these changes may misinterpret them as willful actions instead of unavoidable symptoms that can accompany AD.

Excess Disability. Sometimes the suspiciousness may evolve into delusional or paranoid ideas. These more serious psychological signs reflect maladaptive, unconscious, defensive reactions on the part of the individual in response to the illness. For example, if one repeatedly forgets where one has placed things, one may become very anxious. Some deal with this anxiety poorly and become suspicious that others misplaced or even stole the items. Such responses can deteriorate further with the ill individual fantasizing that a conspiracy is threatening his or her possessions or everyday activities. Changes in neurotransmitter systems and neuropeptides are also likely influencing these symptoms. In addition to the anguish caused by delusions, their further distorting of thought compounds the cognitive impairment of the dementia. Various interventions, including the judicious use of certain medications, can be helpful in these situations (see Chapter 4, page 70).

Mood problems ranging from sadness to deep depression are common. Particularly at the early stage of AD, when the afflicted individual can observe his or her lapses, a depressive reaction can occur. Here, too, deficits along neurotransmitter pathways (especially the biogenic amines that were discussed in Chapter 5) and among neuropeptides are probably playing a part in altered moods. As in the case of delusional thinking, the addition of depression to the dementia of AD can aggravate the person's impairment.

The term used to describe such states of aggravated impairment is "excess disability" (Kahn & Tobin, 1981). Depression, like paranoia, can be treated, and intervention can enable the individual to better cope with the underlying brain disorder. In these situations it is not just a matter of balance between the degree of intellectual deficit on the one side and the level of cognitive capacity on the other that influences patient functioning; it is also a matter of how the nature of an Alzheimer patient's behavior tilts this delicate balance in coping with deficit and drawing upon capacity. One study found 31% of 131 Alzheimer patients to be depressed; upon treatment for their depression, fully 85% showed improvement in terms of mood, activities of daily living, and vegetative (e.g., sleep, appetite, weight) signs (Reifler, Larson, Teri, & Poulsen, 1986).

Moreover, concurrent physical problems from other illnesses that the Alzheimer patient may be experiencing can also produce co-morbidity or excess disability; these compounding general medical problems often respond to clinical intervention as well, thereby lifting some of the patient's added impairment (Larson, Buchner, Uhlmann, & Reifler, 1986; Reifler & Larson, 1988). Overall, the treatment of excess disability states offers one of the most important intervention opportunities available for Alzheimer's disease.

Catastrophic Reaction. As the skills of the individual with AD further deteriorate, the person's frustration threshold also drops. It becomes more common to see a patient react—with marked agitation—to stress, confusion, difficulty with a given task, or failure. The term "catastrophic reaction" is used in such situations where the individual seems to overreact or be disproportionately anxious about everyday challenges, even minor ones such as remembering a phone number or buttoning a shirt (Mace & Rabins, 1981). This can be exasperating and confusing to family and friends who may respond awkwardly by reprimanding the individual for getting so upset. But usually, he or she cannot help it; it is a phenomenon of the illness—a characteristic behavioral manifestation of underlying brain dysfunction. Trying to reduce the stresses in the afflicted individual's environment is often a more productive strategy, one that illustrates the impact that psychological interventions can have on physical aberrations.

Labile Affect. As AD moves toward a later stage, the person with the disorder gradually becomes less aware of his or her growing impairment. To an extent this psychologically protects the ill who are then less overwhelmed emotionally in witnessing their own decline. When a mistake is made, an excuse might be given or responsibility denied. Eventually these ill individuals may experience severe difficulty in remembering basic facts (such as who the President is), what year or month it is, or in recognizing close friends and relatives. With increasing disorientation, there may be trouble finding one's way home. The emotional state of the afflicted may fluctuate widely from moment to moment, from great excitement to irritation to remoteness. Little things may change their mood dramatically—a state called "labile affect." Labile affect has long been recognized as an emotional signal of underlying brain disorder. Yet other individuals, at an advanced stage of the disease, may appear mute and inattentive and have minimal energy.

Final Stage. By the final stage of the disease, many patients become severely regressed in behavior and highly, if not completely, dependent on others for basic care. When the burden on the individual and the family becomes too great and round-the-clock care is called for, it may be necessary to put the patient in a nursing home. Such decisions, even when they are unavoidable or long overdue, commonly stir considerable feelings of guilt and anguish in family members, reflecting the severe psychosocial impact of the brain disorder.

Variations in the Clinical Course. Despite this distressing clinical scenario, symptoms and types of difficulties do differ from person to person with the disorder. The duration alone has enormous variation, lasting for fewer than 3 years with some, and extending to more than 20 with others (Heston, 1983); one might die with the disorder (before reaching the final stage), rather than from it. Even commonly experienced problems vary in sequence, duration, and degree among different patients. Moreover, throughout much of the course of the illness those with AD remain very capable of giving and receiving love, of sharing warm interpersonal relationships, and of participating in a variety of meaningful activities with family and friends. One may no longer be able to do math, but one may still read a magazine with pleasure for months or years to come. Playing the piano for those previously so skilled might become too stressful in the face of increasing mistakes, but singing along with others may for some time still be facile and fun. The chess board may have to be put away, but one's tennis game may stay in there for quite a while. Thus, despite the many exasperating moments there remain many good ones. Challenge, frustration, closeness, sadness, and satisfaction may all be experienced by those who work to help the person with AD cope as best as they can with the illness, and to live through it with dignity. Contemplating the clinical course in this manner is critical to how the practitioner both plans treatment and provides perspective for patient and family alike.

Treating the Patient's Symptoms

Focusing on the classic case described by Alzheimer, one sees the range of symptoms that define the range of treatment strategies that can be mobilized. The following is an excerpt from the November 3, 1906 report that Alois Alzheimer presented at a meeting of the Association of

Southwest German Specialists in Mental Diseases (Alzheimer, 1907; Jarvik & Greenson, 1987):

> The first noticeable symptom of illness shown by this 51-year-old woman was suspiciousness of her husband. Soon, a rapidly increasing memory impairment became evident; she could no longer orient herself in her own dwelling, dragged objects here and there and hid them, and at times, believing that people were out to murder her, started to scream loudly.

As alluded to in the previous chapter, the striking clinical phenomenon about AD is that for a major part of its natural history the predominant signs and symptoms caused by its brain pathology are behavioral as opposed to physical in nature. They are behavioral in the broad sense of the term's meaning, referring to the nature of the patient's cognition, emotional status, psychological state, general behavior, and interpersonal relationships with family and others.

The woman described by Alzheimer in 1906 displayed behavioral problems in all of these areas. Cognition was impaired, as reflected in the description of her "rapidly increasing memory impairment"; emotionally she was distraught to the point of having episodes where she "started to scream loudly"—agitation and/or depression being common in the disorder and contributing to "excess disability"; psychologically, she manifested paranoid delusions that often represent another form of excess disability, in her psychotic concerns that "people were out to murder her"; her general behavior revealed the diminished coping skills ("she could no longer orient herself in her own dwelling") and maladaptive activities (she "dragged objects here and there and hid them") that accompany the progression of the disorder; the psychosocial stress that can emerge in interpersonal relationships and family interactions was portrayed in her manifesting "suspiciousness of her husband."

Regardless of whether the setting is one's home, the community, or a nursing home, these different behavioral symptom clusters can often be alleviated to varying degrees by available treatment strategies. Somatic (e.g., psychopharmacologic drugs) and nonsomatic (e.g., hehavioral and psychotherapeutic interventions) treatment modalities have potential roles at different stages in the course of the disorder—the nonsomatic often alone, at other times in combination with the somatic (Cohen, 1984; Miller & Cohen, 1981; Yesavage & Widrow, 1985).

Behavior as a Window on the Brain. High tech imaging devices are not our only access points for gaining information on what is going on within the brain. By observing behavior, we can gain ideas on where to look or what to look for, in the brain, when something goes wrong.

Observations of behavior can lead to treatment ideas, and at times provide clues as to the nature of underlying brain pathology. The following case example illustrates the point.

Case Example: Mrs. Maret, an 82-year-old widow, illustrated the tendency on the part of many people with marked memory impairment, where their recall of a previous conversation is typically limited or absent—one might find oneself discussing a number of the same things at the next or in several subsequent conversations. I received a lesson from Mrs. Maret one day on how to translate this deficit into a useful intervention. Upon meeting with her that day I arrived at her apartment while she was listening to a cassette from one of her daughters who lived over two thousand miles away. The cassette was of her daughter speaking, and lasted 30 minutes, during which the daughter talked about her latest activities and about those of her own children. Mrs. Maret was thoroughly delighted with the sound of her daughter's voice and the news being related. What was equally interesting was that the tape had arrived nearly a week earlier, and Mrs. Maret had asked her homemaker to play it for her on each of her visits since then. Between playings Mrs. Maret forgot so much of what was said on the tape that each replay seemed to elicit as positive a reaction as if she had just received a new recording.

It occurred to me that this could represent a very useful technique for meaningfully engaging various Alzheimer patients, at certain points in the course of their illness, in a structured, time-filling activity. I began to encourage other families to make tapes with family news, grandchildren singing or performing on instruments, and the like, as a source of appealing, emotionally invested activity for the patient. The main assistance that someone else might have to provide would be to press the play button on the recorder and to rewind the tape. This approach has proved to be very gratifying for the family who participate, satisfying to the patient who benefits from it, and helpful to staff (e.g., in the nursing home setting) in their efforts to engage patients in constructive activities.

This case is somewhat reminiscent of an earlier famous case about H.M., a patient with a long history of seizures and convulsions who was subjected to bilateral surgical removal of the entire region about the hippocampus of his brain in a successful attempt to reduce the frequency and severity of these symptoms (Sagan, 1977). However, the hippocampal disruption caused him to forget everything more than a few hours old. Whatever was told to him one day could be repeated and received on the next day as if it were brand new information. In AD, the hippocampus is noticeably affected along with other parts of the cerebral cortex, revealing a high density of plaques and tangles, and more recently has revealed specific cellular pathology that has been postulated by Hyman and associates to contribute in a highly specific way to the memory disorder in Alzheimer patients (Hyman, Van Hoesen, Damasio, & Barnes, 1984); this might also explain the response of Mrs. Maret to the tape recording. Of course, one does not have to have poor memory to enjoy a story a second time.

From a different vantage point, observations of Mrs. Maret's behavior could have in themselves led the investigator back to the hippocampus, based on the association of the patient's behavior with knowledge of the case of H.M. The findings described by Hyman and associates above would have been waiting to be identified.

In large part, a related scenario led to the identification of the acetylcholine neurotransmitter deficit in AD. Observations by Drachman of AD-like behavior and memory impairment in young subjects taking anticholinergic drugs helped generate the hypothesis of diminished levels of acetylcholine occurring in AD (Drachman & Leavitt, 1974). Similarly, observations of depressive symptomatology and behavior in Alzheimer patients have contributed to the interest in locus coeruleus lesions in AD (Perry & Perry, 1985). The locus coeruleus is the subcortical brain nucleus that is particularly rich in neurons producing the neurotransmitter norepinephrine—a neurotransmitter that has been strongly implicated in mood disorders. Hence, close attention to behavioral phenomena can on occasion suggest clues as to the nature of neuroanatomical and neurochemical changes in brain, as in the case of AD. One's perspective on treatment is then sharpened along both behavioral and biomedical dimensions.

The Treatment of "Excess Disability." While it is recognized that severe depression alone in the elderly can mimic AD, the role of depression in conjunction with the dementia has been less well appreciated. When depression becomes superimposed on top of the dementia, cognitive impairment at that point in the course of the disorder is greater than would otherwise be the case—the state referred to as "excess disability." As emphasized earlier, one of the most important treatment opportunities with Alzheimer patients is the alleviation of excess disability states. At times a most interesting phenomenon is observed when an excess disability state is treated. With the lifting of compounding depression, for example, one might witness an increase in overall functional capacity in the Alzheimer patient at that point in time. Indeed, this can be a rather confusing situation in that one observes actual clinical improvement in the face of an underlying disease process that continues to worsen. Only after further time passes do coping skills again show deterioration. The following case illustrates such a clinical scenario.

Case Example: A 75-year-old brilliant chemist, Professor Janof, was evaluated because of significant trouble he was having with memory and concentration—to the extent that he no longer could balance his checkbook and no longer took an interest in reading. Professor Janof described difficulty noticeable only to him, a year earlier, when he was becoming less facile with complicated equations. To others he still looked quite sharp, but not to himself. This problem was a terrible blow to Professor Janof's self-esteem, and he began to experience trouble sleeping, loss of appetite and weight, and further difficulty concentrating. A thorough differential diagnostic work-up ruled out many causes of dementia-like symptoms that can mimic senile dementia, and left the clinician with the diagnosis of AD. But the impression was that depression was also present. Treatment was instituted for the depression, combining individual psychotherapy and an antidepressant medication. Professor Janof's appetite returned, the weight loss stopped, concentration improved, he started reading again, though trouble with the checkbook continued. The therapeutic work helped Professor Janof come to terms with his underlying disorder, with AD. Residual skills were maximized during that stage in the course of his illness; quality of life during that interval was enhanced.

Without an understanding of the potential for excess disability in the course of AD, Professor Janof may have been denied a treatment opportunity in the face of a diagnosis of AD. But it is the nature of the phenomenon that the patient can show temporary restoration of function while suffering from a progressive illness. As it turned out, Professor Janof had a slowly progressive case of AD. Following the intervention for his depression, another three years passed before he returned to the level of cognitive impairment with which he was first seen clinically. Treatment gave him three better years at a critical juncture in his life course. Diagnostically, the case points out how it is not sufficient to ask "is it depression or is it AD?" One must also question whether it could be both, concurrently. With such recognition one can achieve interim relief for a brain disorder in treating its behavioral overlay.

Delusions can similarly aggravate the course of someone with AD, causing excess disability, and if treated can likewise improve the individual's capacity to deal with his or her environment.

Case Example: Mr. Tursis, a 76-year-old man with AD, who had lost his wife three years earlier, was having increasing difficulty managing his two-bedroom condominium by himself. He had a working daughter and an older sister living in the vicinity, who provided emotional support and help with some of his household responsibilities. However, his increasing incapacity together with the limits on his daughter's time and his sister's strength made it necessary for the family to seek home help for Mr. Tursis. An effort was made to engage the services of a homemaker. At first, Mr. Tursis resisted this idea, saying that he valued his independence and was sure that some stranger would only interfere in his affairs. He finally relented, but the homemaker was allowed to come for only a week, at which point Mr. Tursis told her not to come back. He was defensive about his actions, exclaiming that the homemaker was planning to steal his belongings. Efforts to get him to accept a new homemaker proved futile, and the family wondered whether he would be able to continue living alone under his circumstances; at the same time, Mr. Tursis was very resistant to the idea of moving.

Consultation was sought, and Mr. Tursis consented to have me visit him in his apartment. What emerged during the evaluation, was that in addition to a mild-to-moderate degree of memory impairment and difficulty in following through with various chores, Mr. Tursis also revealed covert paranoid thinking that became apparent only on careful probing. He had subtle but significant concerns about a conspiracy going on among unknown parties, aimed at taking over his holdings. While the delusions were not challenged (which would likely only have provoked the patient at that point and to have caused him to lose confidence in the therapist), the inner tension that he felt about them was real (since both fantasy and reality can stir great anxiety) and was accordingly acknowledged; this became the basis of a therapeutic alliance that permitted him to accept the idea of trying some medication that could help him better cope with the stress of his situation. A small dose of antipsychotic medication was prescribed in conjunction with follow-up supportive psychotherapeutic visits. The delusions subsided, and Mr. Tursis allowed the idea of homemaker assistance to be brought up again. This time he was able to tolerate a stranger coming into his home, and the arrangement worked out. Despite gradual further deterioration of memory and cognitive functions, Mr. Tursis was able to remain in his apartment because of the homemaker's help. Mr. Tursis died four years later, from a heart attack, at home.

The case illustrates several points. It shows the great degree to which delusions can compound coping capacity in AD; it shows what improvement can follow if these delusions can be lifted or lightened. A sense of what brings on the delusions might be inferred. While a biological basis for delusions in AD is offered as a factor of alterations in neurotransmitter levels and in the synchronism of their actions, psychological explanations are also postulated. The individual with AD is suffering severe losses. As one's intellectual capacity to examine these losses becomes impaired, one's mind might begin working in psychodynamically defensive ways, making one think that the problems are not internal, but external—not with oneself, but with others (Verwoerdt, 1981). Such emotional turmoil might then reach delusional proportions with paranoid thinking. This case also illustrates how with varying durations to the clinical course of AD in different individuals, one might die *with* the disease (from other causes) at a less advanced stage, rather than *from* it (as many have suggested) at an advanced stage.

Delusions accompanying AD can also contribute to a situation of "triple jeopardy" in a family feeling overwhelmed in their efforts to help a loved one afflicted with the disorder at home. The first part of the triple jeopardy is the family experiencing the emotional anguish of watching someone close to them suffer the illness. The second part is the physical and emotional burden the family experiences in providing care for this individual. If the patient then develops delusions focused on the family (as in the case of Alois Alzheimer's patient who angrily accused her husband of having affairs), then these emotional assaults against those already anguished and burdened might become simply too overwhelming for the family to be able to still deal with the patient at home. An alternative placement might then become necessary. But if the delusions can be brought under control, then the resiliency of the family might be restored, and their capacity to continue to help the patient at home strengthened. In such a scenario the concept of excess disability can be appreciated in how it can apply to the family as well—where they become subject to stresses which can respond to treatment focused on both the patient and the family.

Similar excess disability states can be seen in elderly patients with other forms of dementia, particularly with strokes or multi-infarct dementia. Depression and delusions can compound the cognitive impairment in these patients as well, and similarly respond to treatments that alleviate suffering, increase coping capacities, and lessen family burden.

It should also be recognized that excess disability in the Alzheimer patient can result from concomitant physical problems as well as accompanying emotional ones. It is common for the elderly in general to have more than one chronic illness. Thus, the Alzheimer patient with poorly controlled congestive heart failure will have a more difficult time with both diseases. Better control of the cardiac disorder would likely lead to improved overall functioning for this individual.

The Treatment of Memory Dysfunction. The search for memory enhancing agents continues with excitement mounting, but as discussed in the previous chapter, this excitement is found within the research community with an eye to the future—not within the practice community with the needs of the present. More than 20 categories of pharmacologic agents have been tried for the treatment of cognitive impairment in Alzheimer's disease (Funkenstein, Hicks, Dysken, & Davis, 1981; Reisberg, 1983). These have included the cholinergic drugs (including choline, lecithin, and physostigmine, and THA which remain at the research stage) discussed in Chapter 6 (pp. 127–128), procaine hydrochloride (Gerovital-H3®) reviewed in Chapter 10 (p. 211), vasodilators, vitamins, stimulants, anticoagulants, and many more. Unfortunately, no drug has demonstrated clear efficacy, though a few medicines have had some equivocally positive results in patients at the initial stage of AD; this group includes the dihydroergotoxine mesylate (Hydergine®) and piracetam (Nootropil®)—reports on both drugs being similar. Since Hydergine is the most extensively used drug in efforts to alleviate cognitive impairment, the following summary of studies on it is provided (Yesavage, 1983):

> Dihydroergotoxine mesylate is the most widely prescribed medication for the indication of dementia worldwide. Nevertheless, clinicians remain skeptical of its clinical effects. However, at least 22 double-blind placebo controlled studies have shown it to be superior to placebo in this indication. Skeptics argue that the medication may improve some psychological tests inconsistently across studies but that the perceived improvements remain quite small. Optimists argue that any change seen in such populations is welcome. Ongoing research is examining the use of higher doses of the medication, as well as the combination of medication with psychotherapy. (p. 377)

Others question whether Hydergine "actually acts by improving mood and lessening anxiety, thus improving test performance that was depressed for emotional reasons" (Funkenstein et al., 1981); in this regard, it would not be having a primary memory enhancing effect, but one not dissimilar to improvements observed in excess disability states of AD.

A fundamental distinction to keep in mind concerning the use of drugs for treating the symptoms of AD is that there are two very different categories of drugs to consider. On the one hand, there are those drugs—mostly experimental—used in attempts to modify the underlying memory impairment; on the other hand, there are those drugs—psychotropic medications already in use—that are prescribed to alleviate the excess disability states of depression and delusions that compound underlying cognitive dysfunction in AD (Goodnick, Gershon, & Salzman, 1984). Although efficacy with the first category of drugs is not yet clinically impressive, success with the second group of medications is much more apparent. The opportunity for a positive impact on excess disability with the second group of drugs can be seen in the above cases of Professor Janof (where an antidepressant was used) and Mr. Tursis (where an antipsychotic was prescribed).

While we wait for more effective drugs in the treatment of cognitive impairment, we nonetheless have at hand a variety of behavioral interventions which can provide memory patches or crutches to those suffering intellectual decline. There are a host of memory training strategies and information organizing aids that can be drawn upon, ranging from simple notes as reminders to more sophisticated clinical approaches. The effect of these behavioral interventions is often much more dramatic than any of the drug effects to date (Eisdorfer, Cohen, & Preston, 1981; Yesavage & Widrow, 1985; Zarit, Cole, & Guider, 1981).

Case Example: An evaluation was requested on an 80-year-old widow, with the impression that placement in a nursing home would be necessary. The woman, Mrs. Adrian, was living alone in an independent-living apartment building for older adults. She had a son and a daughter who would call her regularly to see how she was doing, and drop by as necessary to assist with grocery shopping and related needs. Mrs. Adrian had been experiencing slowly worsening memory difficulties over the past couple of years, and more recently had begun to wander from her apartment, particularly in the evening. It was the wandering that had become especially worrisome to her family and neighbors, who feared that she would get lost or be harmed; they felt that because of the wandering, Mrs. Adrian would no longer be able to live by herself in her apartment. A comprehensive evaluation was carried out, and an earlier tentative diagnosis of AD appeared to have been correct.

Consultation with the family proved very interesting in that an intriguing theme emerged at different times in the son's and daughter's descriptions of their mother. More with a fondness than with a patronizing tone they described their mother as having gone through life as a good "sheep," always following the recommendations of responsible authority figures. Thinking about this characterization, I wondered if Mrs. Adrian was so responsive to authoritative instructions, might she follow such advice written out on a large note to be attached to the inside of her door. I recommended that we tape onto her apartment door a large prescription that would read "please do not leave your apartment after 5:00 P.M. in the evening." It was with some amusement and skepticism that the family participated in this effort. But to the awe of all, this behavioral strategy had a major impact on Mrs. Adrian's wandering. Checking with the neighbors during the first few weeks after placing the note on the door, we learned that the wandering had diminished noticeably, and the general concern about Mrs. Adrian's safety had greatly abated.

Other behavioral strategies were also employed. Some housekeeping assistance was arranged, not only to help with chores around the apartment, but also to provide more structure to Mrs. Adrian's daily routine. In addition, most of her medications were able to be rearranged so as to be taken once or twice a day, which allowed the son and daughter to develop a system of one of them calling each morning and evening to remind their mother to take her medicine, and staying on the phone until she did so.

In this manner, memory patches were devised that were sufficiently effective so as to allow Mrs. Adrian to remain in her apartment (to which she was very attached) for another two years, at which point it became apparent that she needed to be in a more protective environment. But the behavioral interventions had added two years to Mrs. Adrian's strong desire to live independently.

Two of the biggest factors that influence nursing home placement—wandering and medication management—had been effectively controlled with thoughtful, straightforward behavioral approaches.

This case illustrates not only the potential role and efficacy of behavioral approaches, but also the value of taking a careful history in order to understand how an individual's life-long patterns and personality traits might relate to treatment planning.

Treatment at the Late Stage of AD and Related Disorders. Whereas the opportunity for treatment in general for AD and related disorders is underappreciated, the ability to treat the patient at the late stage of disorder is even less recognized. Even when patients have severe cognitive impairment there are clinical interventions that can have an important effect on the interactions between them and significant others. In long-term care settings where many individuals with AD and related disorders have marked dementia, one of the most important needs is for the staff to get to know the patients. This can be a serious problem because of a patient's memory dysfunction and difficulty in giving a history. The clinician who is familiar with the patient's background can, through consultation, make a major contribution in helping the patient better adjust to the new environment, while assisting the staff in developing a more relevant treatment plan. The following case example reflects such a situation.

Case Example: Mrs. Crawford, an 80-year-old childless widow, was seen because of a recurrence of depression. She had a fair degree of insight into the genesis of her disorder, recognizing a relationship between dark moods and dreams of having been scapegoated for family difficulties by her father. From early childhood she had distinguished herself in many ways, from ice skating, to good looks, to excellent job performance. But her father never seemed to recognize her achievements—instead, found minor faults to criticize. Nonetheless, she was proud of her interesting experiences and accomplishments and took much satisfaction in describing them to me and in registering my positive reactions.

As a young woman, while living in Hollywood, she had competed for beaus with some of the early starlets of the silver screen. She and Mary Pickford got involved with the same man; Mrs. Crawford lost in that competition. She eventually married and settled into a steady white-collar job. By age 65 she was a widow and felt she wanted a basic change in life. Always having been an outstanding driver, she took a job which she described as a "chauffeur for rich ladies." Here, as in all her activities, she mustered up great energy and devotion. To protect these "fine women" she decided to clandestinely "pack a pistol." She continued this work for about five years before going into retirement again.

Then at age 75, experiencing some financial strain, she relied once more on her diverse skills and resourcefulness and turned to the game of poker with considerable success among another circle of "rich ladies." By age 80 she had returned to retired life, spending increasing time with a new boyfriend. But shortly thereafter she lost the intimacy and companionship of this very dear friend through his death. Feeling suddenly alone she began to review her disappointments in life, instead of her many satisfying experiences. The depression that gradually developed eventually led to her seeking out a psychiatrist. Her depression finally lifted several months later when she struck up a close relationship with another man. She giggled over her awareness of a general pattern she displayed in choosing close male companions; for the most part they were older men, and she wondered whether this reflected longstanding attempts to somehow resolve the ambivalent feelings she still had for her father. Her most recent romance was to be no exception, as she began dating a 97-year-old man. With the continued remission of her depression we terminated therapy.

Three years later I received most distressing news. Mrs. Crawford had suffered a major stroke, leaving her severely demented, with cognitive impairment similar to that of an advanced stage of AD. I went to see her in the nursing home. When I arrived I was stunned with what I witnessed. Rather than the center of attraction she had always been, she was now looked on as a source of irritation. Her intellectual dysfunction, agitation, and high level of disability had made her quite difficult to manage. I was also struck by the matter-of-factness with which staff passed by her with minimal visual contact—in such contrast to the attention she had commanded throughout life.

The double tragedy experienced by the patient in relation to her history and her identity became apparent. The first tragedy was more obvious—the distance, the break from her own history, from her own past, due to marked memory impairment. The second, less obvious, tragedy was the distance she experienced from others due to their separation from her, because of their inability to know about the interesting history she could no longer convey. (In this regard, we all have a compound history, a two-faceted history—a history of ourselves as we know it and a history of ourselves as others know it. Not to be known by others, to be in effect without a history by being unable to relate one's past, puts a person at a severe disadvantage in eliciting the understanding and empathy of others; a competitive edge of the human condition has been lost. This is the plight of many patients with dementia, with AD.) Mrs. Crawford had lost much of the appeal ordinarily derived from others having known her and about her life experiences. Here, the clinician can be enormously helpful in conveying the individual's personal and dynamic history, his or her clinical biography.

An attempt was then made to restore some of this competitive edge, this most interesting human phenomenon—one's history, one's biography. Scrapbooks, photos, news clippings, and other personal items of memorabilia were gathered in the process of trying to dynamically portray a sense of Mrs. Crawford's past to the staff. The impact was pronounced. When I returned the next week there was considerably more verbal and nonverbal engagement between the staff and the patient. And as more time passed it became apparent that in addition to the staff feeling more in touch with the patient because of their being more in touch with her personal history, fragments of disjointed thoughts she would express were somewhat better understood due to the enlarged frame of reference in which they were heard. Though the magnitude of dementia was not altered, the patient's agitation was reduced and her connection with others enhanced; quality of life improved.

The problem of imparting a patient's history though is more complicated than what has been described. This is because of the dual problem of there being more than one shift of personnel during the course of each day and substantial staff turnover (a particular problem with nursing assistants at nursing homes) during the course of the year.

How then can one convey a patient's history in a practical manner for each shift and for ongoing new staff? Certainly it is difficult to achieve this effect with a typical chart history; the length alone might discourage many from reading it. One could take advantage of audio and video technology and record the history on audio or video cassettes. Some institutions would have the resources to develop a program of audiovisual histories, while for those settings where the costs might be prohibitive, audio cassette histories could still be feasible. Staff on all shifts might be much more likely to obtain these histories because of ease of access— listening to or watching a cassette presentation as opposed to pondering over a chart. Such a process could also facilitate case conferences or dialogue about the patient among staff viewing or listening to the tapes at the same time.

Family members could also assume an important role here and would probably derive much satisfaction by contributing to the information and presentation on the cassettes. Especially if a given family member is a good story teller, that person should be involved in giving the patient's biography. The experience could be rewarding all the way around. From this case example it might be appreciated that in patients with severe dementia, the role of biography can be as important as that of biology in the overall approach to treatment.

Intervening with Significant Others

The case of Mrs. Crawford not only illustrates the opportunity to clinically intervene at an advanced stage of dementia, it also points out the need to focus on significant others as to how they can influence the patient's clini cal course in a helpful or hindering manner. In addition to examining the effect that significant others have on the patient, it is equally important to be aware of the effect that the patient has on significant others, particularly on caregiving relatives (Brody, 1986; Haley, Levine, Brown, Berry, & Hughes, 1987). Clinical depression and anxiety on the part of family members is disturbingly prevalent, with some startling reports indicating that as many as 80% of spousal caregivers are so affected at some point during the course of AD (Gallagher, 1987). On the positive side, caregivers appear to respond very well to a variety of intervention programs, ranging from family support groups to professional consultations. Hence, for patient and family alike, AD represents a major public health problem, but one where there are important therapeutic openings for both.

The case example below illustrates both the anguish that family members can experience with an inadequate understanding of AD, and the help that can be provided to both patient and family through a treatment plan focusing on the family system as a whole. It also deals with one of the great frustrations many family members experience when they visit relatives with AD or a related disorder in the nursing home—finding what to say or trying to make conversation with someone extremely impaired in their ability to verbally communicate. One of the pioneers in geriatric psychiatry experienced this dilemma with his own mother and was inspired to write a classic paper entitled "What Do You Say to Your Mother When You Have Nothing to Say?" (Weinberg, 1974).

Case Example: The son of a 74-year-old woman living in a nursing home requested consultation on how to deal with the anguish he was feeling in not being able to effectively engage in conversations with his mother. He described that if he asked her a question, she would usually not be able to answer it, while rarely raising questions for him to answer and no longer inquiring about his own family. When his 14-year-old daughter visited her grandmother in the nursing home, she was distraught over this same pattern, having mistakenly personalized it in thinking that her beloved grandmother was no longer interested in the granddaughter's activities.

The nature of his mother's memory and cognitive deficits was explained to the son. He was told how both recent and remote memory with his mother were impaired, that she had great difficulty on her own in connecting new ideas coming in with fragments of stored memories, thereby making it difficult for her to sustain conversation for very long on the same topic without drifting into some other area or else into silence. It was explained that without very careful attention to visitors structuring the conversation, interchange would be very limited. Visitors needed to recognize that they would have to be more active in providing topics and not expecting well developed responses. It was recommended that the granddaughter, for example, bring in a school yearbook, and start turning the pages and talking about the different people and activities going on. In this way, the granddaughter would be helped in "knowing what to say." Conversation would be easier to sustain, and this structure would make it easier for the grandmother to respond within her capacity to do so. Such an approach, it was pointed out, would provide structure for patient and visitor alike, and facilitate the goal of sharing company and time.

It was also pointed out that sharing meaningful time did not necessarily require that conversation would always have to be taking place. When people go to a movie or a concert together, conversation is not even appropriate during performances that can last 2 to 3 hours. In the nursing home, music can be listened to quietly together, or nature walks or rides can be taken with long intervals of silent enjoyment of the environment.

Addressing the Patient's Environment

The interaction of the patient with his or her environment needs to be addressed not only in psychosocial terms, but in a physical context as well (Lawton, 1981). From one perspective, supportive and facilitating aspects of the environment require understanding; from a different vantage point, stressful and safety threatening elements in one's surroundings demand consideration. Clinical course can be profoundly influenced by either parameter.

Because of cognitive impairment individuals with AD becomes less able to negotiate their everyday environment. Hence, their environment becomes more stressful, raising the risk of "catastrophic reactions" (see earlier discussion of this phenomenon). Threats to safety enter here as well for the Alzheimer patient. For example, forgetting which way to turn at a stairway might lead to a fall and fractures, or not remembering to turn off the oven could lead to other adverse consequences. A careful study of the environment could help identify a number of potential risks to personal safety and other factors that could cause frustration and therefore extra stress.

Thoughtful approaches to creatively restructuring the environments of these individuals could easily pay off in terms of not only improving their sense of well-being, but in increasing their basic capacity to remain in the community. Such efforts could include the use of cues or signs reminding one to turn off the stove or to lock the door; movement of one's bedroom from an upper floor to a lower one to avoid additional stairways to stumble down during nighttime wandering; the involvement of a helper to assist in shopping to prevent frustration from forgetting essential groceries or from trouble in finding the way back home. Some of these approaches were taken in the earlier case example of Mrs. Adrian. There is a growing literature of advice on many practical matters of this nature in helping Alzheimer patients through the everyday trials of their illness (Cohen & Eisdorfer, 1986; Heston & White, 1983; Mace & Rabins, 1981). Also important to recognize is that the value of examining what is stressful or facilitating in the environment applies to institutional (e.g., nursing home) settings as much as community sites (Lawton, 1981).

Reviewing the Role of the Service System

All of the elements delineated in the initial treatment planning outline apply to community and institutional settings alike, whether the focus is on diagnosis, clinical course, patient symptomatology, significant others, or environment (Brody, 1981; Gaitz & Samorajski, 1985; Kahn & Tobin, 1981). AD is a complex problem. A comprehensive clinical approach to it is not simple. But a treatment plan that makes a difference is feasible. An effective treatment plan will reflect understanding of the different problems that accompany AD, knowledge of a range of intervention strategies, awareness of the diversity of available service sites and providers (from both formal and informal support systems), and appreciation of how best to coordinate efforts at different points in time during the natural history of the disorder.

Examining Social Policy

It would be incomplete to end a discussion on interventions without reflecting on the role of social policy (Binstock, 1985; Estes, 1988; U.S. Congress, Office of Technology Assessment, 1987). Certainly the most dramatic way to resolve the mounting crisis in care and costs that surrounds AD is to have a major breakthrough in research leading to the cure or prevention of the disorder. Short of this, research findings that could translate into treatment to arrest the disorder if not reverse it would also represent a profound contribution. While research on AD is burgeoning in the United States, the resources allocated to it have been relatively small—a situation not at all helped by the serious economic state of the nation. It is perhaps provocative to note that the money devoted to research on AD in 1980 (about $10 million), represented a mere 0.05% (five one-hundredths of one percent) of that year's $20 billion dollars going into nursing homes, a setting so heavily populated with Alzheimer patients. By 1988 the research budget for the disorder had risen to about $95 million. But most agree that the magnitude of the problem dwarfs these dollar amounts.

To begin with, the social policy agenda for AD will have to reexamine the amount of research support our society can make available. But while we are waiting for the fruits of this research, we must deal with the present approximately two million patients and families with AD—a number that will grow with the doubling of the elderly population over the next 50 years. Hence, while waiting for a cure, there is a list of social policy questions that relate to care—to the need and ability to provide a range of useful interventions and services now. Such questions could address the enhancement of services in the community that are presently assisting families in caring for loved ones with AD at home, the evolution of health and long-term care insurances to improve access to these services as well as to alternative living arrangements, quality of care issues in the nursing home, and further study in all of these areas. This should be a broad national agenda, not just a federal initiative. It is a job for government and the private sector together, one that can best be accomplished through the collaboration of both.

Hippocrates once pointed out that "extreme remedies are very appropriate for extreme diseases." In the case of AD, a long time passed before it was recognized as a disease—its extreme impact on the individual, the family, and society having been somehow dismissed as a cruel fate due to the aging of the brain. But with the recognition of AD as a disorder, the quest for remedies has only recently begun to have any semblance to Hippocrates' age-old prescription. And it must be stressed that the aging brain is not without its own resources and capacities. These will be discussed in some detail in Part III.

III

Capacities of the Aging Brain

8

Resiliency and Repair of the Aging Brain

It had been long thought and taught that after development of the brain was completed early in life, the organ functioned like a "static, 'hard-wired' machine" (Shepherd, 1983). Never mind that the idea of potential repair for damaged brain tissue had difficulty finding the light of day; the concept of modifiability or adaptability per se of brain function seemed equally foreign—all of this despite everyday knowledge from behavioral research that our stores of information and skills grow over time and that our patterns of emotional response reflect the influence of experience. It was as if mind and personality had no relationship to the organic substrate we know of as the brain. Those who recognized that behavior was not rigid and that it had to be influenced by an inner environment as well as an outer one began to explore for comparable "plasticity" on the part of the central nervous system. The basic functional and anatomical unit of the brain that investigators focused on was the nerve cell involved in higher mental functions, also known as the *neuron* (see Figure 2.3).

The neuron consists of a number of structural components, including: a *cell body* that contains the *nucleus,* the latter housing the nucleic acids DNA and RNA which are involved in the transmission of genetic information to control the synthesis of protein for the nerve cell as a whole (the term nucleus is used in another context, as well, to describe certain dense groupings of nerve cells in various parts of the brain); *dendrites,* which are branching fibers receiving impulses from other neurons and conducting impulses to the cell body of the host neuron; *dendritic spines,* which are tiny thorn-like projections from a dendrite, the spines themselves serving as impulse receivers; *axons,* which transmit impulses away from the cell body to the dendrites of other neurons; and *neurofibers,* thin fibrils more within the axon than either the cell body or dendrites of the neuron, implicated in the transmission of impulses. The impulses between neurons are conveyed by a variety of chemicals known as *neurotransmitters;* the juncture between the transmitting axon of one neuron and the receiving dendrite of another is known as the *synapse,* while the actual space a neurotransmitter must cross is referred to as the *synaptic cleft.* A single neuron may be involved in thousands of synaptic connections, given the number of dendrites and dendritic spines it may possess (Kaplan & Saddock, 1980). Meanwhile, it is estimated that there are over 15 billion neurons in the brain. Considering the number of connections possible for a single neuron, the number of possibilities for intercommunication among the 15 billion is truly awesome.

However, the problem with neurons is that if something destroys them (e.g., trauma or disease), the brain does not generate new ones. Moreover, by age 2, development of cells within the brain is nearly complete, with little if any formation of new nerve cells thereafter. The inability of the brain to generate new neurons in response to loss of nerve cells *and* the lack of development of additional neurons after the first few years of life differentiate brain tissue from so many other tissues of the body. These two limitations on neurons explain why brain disease is so serious; they also have influenced many to regard the brain as lacking plasticity.

In contrast, if one loses blood, the bone marrow generates new red blood cells—a process that continues throughout the life cycle. Similarly, with skin and liver, turnover and generation of new cells is an ongoing process. Skin cells can be destroyed in an abrasion, only to be replaced by newly generated cells that leave no trace of the earlier injury; this is why skin is so responsive to *plastic* surgery. Given the difference with neurons, does this mean that the brain has no restorative capacity—no potential for plasticity?

PLASTICITY OF THE AGING BRAIN

Even though the number of brain cells does not increase after the first few years, brain weight continues to rise for a couple of decades. One can conclude, therefore, that the anatomy of the brain is *not* static. Cell bodies of neurons undoubtedly expand in size, and dendrites both in length and number, to partially explain this weight gain. More dendrites means more interconnections between neurons and probably improved as well as more complicated functions. The ongoing capacity of neurons to generate new dendrites represents one component of the brain plasticity counterpart to behavioral plasticity (Cotman & Holets, 1985). Thus, while the brain fails to generate new neurons beyond the initial complement, existing neurons can adapt to increase the number and perhaps the nature of their communications (Brody, 1987).

If a neuron is damaged it does have some regenerative capacity, but only if its cell body remains viable; otherwise, the nerve cell dies. An intact cell body permits a damaged neuron to regenerate an axon as well as dendrites. In cases of brain damage where various neurons are destroyed, proximal surviving neurons respond with the generation of additional dendrites from their cell bodies in an effort to compensate for the intercellular connections disrupted as a result of the lost nerve cells. The term used to describe this process is "compensatory dendritic sprouting." The aging brain's capacity to maintain an adequate circuitry among viable nerve cells is an important determinant of its resiliency. When the adequacy of this circuitry is challenged by the normal loss of neurons over time and by the exaggerated loss from disease, remaining neurons respond with efforts to expand their architecture. Axons and dendrites comprise a major portion of a neuron's architecture. Scientists theorize that to the extent this architecture can be elaborated—as with compensatory dendritic sprouting—the richness of the circuitry may be maintained among the healthy, and partially restored among the ill (Cotman & Holets, 1985).

In addition to anatomical variations in the mature brain, there are chemical adaptations as well, thereby expanding the repertoire of responses that can play a part in brain plasticity (Carlsson, 1985b). It is important to examine these adaptations not only in reaction to damage, but in response to positive stimuli as well. There have been a number of attempts, for example, to study the impact of enriched environments on brain plasticity. Researchers have wondered whether mental exercise exerts an effect on brain tissue similar to that of physical exercise on muscles. The results of several such studies have been fascinating, and even more so when the brain studied was an aging one.

The Effect of a Mentally Stimulating Environment on the Aging Brain

During the mid-1960s, a series of experiments was designed to study the impact of challenging and stimulating environments on the brains of rats. Clearly rat brains and human brains are not equivalent, but animal models have long had their place in the history of medicine in generating hypotheses, pointing to new directions, and leading to breakthroughs in better understanding health and illness in man. The mid-1960s studies described a number of interesting changes in the brains of rats placed in enriched laboratory environments. The cerebral cortex or thinking part of the brains of these rats was found after such stimulation to have thickened, to have increased in weight, and to have contained greater activity of the enzyme acetylcholinesterase (which affects the metabolism of the neurotransmitter acetylcholine believed to be involved in memory and intellectual function) (Diamond, Krech, & Rosenberg, 1964; Diamond, 1983). The researchers also found that there were more glial cells in these brains. *Glial cells* (their name derived from the Greek word meaning glue) are believed to carry out a number of auxiliary metabolic functions to assist neurons. They are viewed as being involved in the transport of active substances between capillaries and neurons, in the formation of the fatty sheath that insulates the axon of the neuron, and in affecting various enzymatic activities that influence neuronal functions.

The enriched environments produced changes in neurons of the rat brains as well. Though the number of neurons was not affected, both the cell bodies and the nuclei of these neurons demonstrated increases in size, suggesting enhanced metabolic activity within the neurons. A further change of note was an increase in the dendritic spines on the cortical neurons of the experimental animals, suggesting heightened communication among the nerve cells. Age was also considered in this research. It was found that an enriched environment produced as great an increase in brain weight in fully mature rats as it did in young rats, although the adult rats required a longer period of environmental stimulation to show the maximum effect.

Subsequent research by Diamond (1983) on enriched environments focused more intensively on aged rats. Results found with young rats were replicated with aging ones. Findings revealed, too, that terminal dendrites of neurons in positively stimulated old rats were significantly longer than comparable dendrites in other old rats not subjected to more challenging environmental stimuli. Again, the alteration in dendritic architecture raised the idea of improved communications among existing neurons.

Another interesting finding from the enriched environment research related to a pigment known as *lipofuscin,* which accumulates with aging in brain cells of rats and humans alike (Diamond, 1983). One of the theories of aging hypothesizes that the build-up of lipofuscin influences the aging process (these theories will be further discussed in Chapter 10). Diamond reported that there was less lipofuscin in the cerebral cortex of aged rats exposed to enriched environments as compared to control animals, though the differences were found to be not statistically significant enough to reach any conclusions or to base any hypotheses.

It should now be apparent that concepts of brain plasticity are relevant to both health and illness perspectives on the aging brain (Franzen &

Sullivan, 1987). The idea of resiliency applies to development on the one hand, and repair on the other. From a disorder vantage point, disease or injury to the brain results in attempted reparative responses—via regeneration of dendrites or axons from damaged neurons, as well from compensatory sprouting of surviving neurons in response to the destruction of neighboring nerve cells. From a developmental perspective, experience or environmental enrichment induces related anatomical variations in the neuron and its intercellular milieu. Though the magnitude of health promotion and clinical potential that these central nervous system response capacities hold for the human aging brain remains to be determined, they point to new frontiers for research. The influence of man's environment on the aging brain gains serious new attention. So, too, does the potential for resiliency and repair of damaged aging brain tissue, with new evidence coming from burgeoning human as well as animal studies (Cotman & Nieto-Sampedro, 1984; Freed, de Medinaceli, & Wyatt, 1985; Schneider, 1979).

While most of this discussion has addressed anatomical aspects of brain plasticity, neurochemical considerations also are highly significant. The influence of chemistry on morphology is dramatically illustrated in the action of hormones; witness the pronounced effect of hormones on the structure of both internal and external bodily organs during puberty and menopause. Discoveries of diverse and powerfully active brain chemicals continue to emerge from the burgeoning arenas of neuroscience research. Such discoveries add to our understanding of certain aging brain phenomena, and generate hypotheses to explain others. Research on neurotransmitters, for example, has linked an acetylcholine deficiency to Alzheimer's disease (see Chapter 7). Studies of the neuroendocrine system have generated a search for brain hormones functioning like clocks that control the aging process (see Chapter 10). Investigations of neurotrophic substances have provided new insights into plasticity of the aging brain.

Neurotrophic Substances and the Aging Brain

Neurotrophic substances have been receiving increasing attention as to their effect on plasticity and repair in young and old brains alike, including more recent attention to their potential role in altering the course of Alzheimer's disease. *Trophic* comes from the Greek word meaning nutritive. A variety of chemical agents that affect membranes and structural components of neurons are under study for their trophic properties. Their ability to influence enzyme activity and growth of nerve cells is also of considerable interest. Best known among these chemicals is nerve growth factor (NGF), a protein molecule apparently produced within the central nervous system, with some structural similarities to insulin (Shepherd, 1983).

Different lines of investigation are under way with NGF. Its ability to induce dendritic sprouting and the growth of axons is being examined by a number of investigators (Freed, de Medinaceli, & Wyatt, 1985). Other studies have found that NGF has increased the level of activity of the enzyme choline acetyltransferase (ChAT) in the brains of rats (Mobley, Rutkowski, Tennekoon, Buchanan, & Johnson, 1985). ChAT has been the focus of a large body of research on the aging brain in recent years because of the enzyme's involvement in the synthesis of acetylcholine, the neurotransmitter most consistently found to have a major role in memory function. Furthermore, studies on Alzheimer's disease have repeatedly found diminished levels of both ChAT and acetylcholine in the brains of victims of this disorder. Hence, preliminary findings of NGF causing increased ChAT activity are of note because of the potential relevance to research on maintaining memory function and to research on treating Alzheimer's disease.

Two other findings about NGF are relevant in planning further research (Mobley et al., 1985). The first pertains to the mode of administering NGF. When NGF was administered peripherally in the neck by subcutaneous injection, no change in ChAT activity was found; direct administration into the fluid chambers of the brain by an intracerebroventricular approach was the effective mode of application. Secondly, other investigations have found that "damaged" cholinergic neurons (the nerve cells that produce acetylcholine) appear to be more sensitive to NGF than intact neurons. This latter finding makes the potential role of NGF in disease states all the more intriguing as a research question.

Nerve growth factor is not the only neurotrophic agent capturing the curiosity of aging brain investigators (Freed et al., 1985). Another substance promoting growth of neuronal processes is referred to as "heart-conditioned medium." It contains chemicals extracted from culture medium upon which heart tissue has been kept alive. Like NGF, heart-conditioned medium has trophic effects on cholinergic neurons, elevating ChAT activity. Animal studies have found it to not only stimulate axonal and dendritic elaboration, but nerve cell survival as well. Ultimately, the goal of research on neurotrophic factors is to discover trophic agents that have the capacity to enhance the brain's recuperative powers—substances that theoretically might act by catalyzing and better regulating the above neural regenerative capacities, by triggering latent but yet to be discovered regeneration mechanisms in the central nervous system, by overcoming the effects of yet to be discovered mechanisms inhibiting brain tissue regeneration, or by a combination of all these processes. In looking at the development of the brain over the ages, one wonders what potentials derived from a lengthy evolution lie hidden, latent, and retrievable in the human brain, including the human brain as it ages.

New Frontiers of Research

The preliminary nature of the above experiments and findings needs to be kept in mind. They remain largely in the realm of research, not practice. But this is not to minimize their significance, for they are already pointing to exciting and potentially promising new directions of inquiry. They also join a history of biological research that has been bringing us closer to grasping some of the fundamental elements and processes that shape the way life unfolds—from the not-that-long-ago discovered structure and function of DNA to yet elusive mechanisms that influence our development, behavior, and aging. Ultimately we may find ourselves at the doorstep of understanding how a single cell (an ovum), with its particular complement of DNA, can eventually differentiate into a highly specialized organism with many organ systems and multibillions of cells. If so, we may come to know how to better trigger regenerative processes within the brain. Conversely, studies of resiliency and repair of the brain may lead us to new insights into physiological growth and development in general. In the process of probing the brain, of uncovering previously unrecognized anatomical and physiological events, secrets of our most mysterious organ are becoming unlocked. Research on the aging brain is both adding to and benefiting from these landmark developments. The aging brain offers us a different door through which to come into contact with many of the extraordinary factors that affect health and illness of the organism as a whole. This frontier is opening up very fast.

BRAIN GRAFTS AND AGING

The year was 1979, and the achievement was extraordinary. In a landmark collaborative experiment involving scientists at the National Institute of Mental Health in the U.S. and at the Karolinska Institute in Stockholm, the first demonstration of functional brain transplants occurred (Perlow et al., 1979). A Parkinson's disease simulating lesion was created within the brain of a host rat. Parkinson's disease, largely a disease of later life, is associated with a deficiency of the neurotransmitter dopamine which is produced by neurons in the substantia nigra, a subcortical nucleus (group of nerve cells) found in the midbrain (see Figure 2.1). In this experiment, the lesion was created in the substantia nigra. Intact tissue from the corresponding part of the brain of a donor rat was then carefully excised, and a graft was attempted. Two remarkable events followed. First, the graft took. Second, the transplanted tissue began to carry out its chemical function of producing dopamine and succeeded in reducing the motor abnormalities of the experimentally induced parkinsonian state. Until then talk about brain grafts more typically evoked images of Frankenstein, the macabre, science fiction, even horror. Suddenly, a new sense of hope for the repair of damaged and diseased brains gained legitimacy—couched with caution about the considerably further distance this research had to travel and about the ethical issues involved. The relevance to the elderly is clear.

Research on Brain Grafts

Brain graft research is important in its own terms. It is important, too, as an example of cutting edge research that stirs significant scientific curiosity and comparable ethical concerns. Many of the new frontiers of biological research on aging may well elicit this same mixture of reactions.

Current brain graft research focuses primarily on anatomical sites of brain tissue that have a specific chemical producing function. The focus is on grafting particular groups of brain cells, not on transplanting the entire brain as in the fictional case of Frankenstein.

New frontiers are forever fraught with fears and uncertainties, but a background of hope often fuels great benefits for mankind. The potential applications of neural transplants to the aging brain fit into this consideration. Since that 1979 turning point report of grafted neurons being capable of bringing about appropriate neurochemical and behavioral responses under the control of the host brain, research on neural transplantation has been dramatically on the rise. Where general concepts of brain plasticity have succeeded in cracking the seemingly impervious armor of ignorance that made the brain seem immutable, brain graft studies have put a huge hole in it.

Brief History of Brain and Neural Transplants

Scientific efforts aimed at neural transplantation date back to 1890 (Gash, Collier, & Sladek, 1985). It was not until 1962, though, that the area attracted major attention through the startling experiments by the Russian surgeon Demikhov who reported successfully transplanting the upper part of one dog's body (including the head) to another dog. The host animals apparently survived only brief periods of time, none longer than a month. Then in 1965, a different team of scientists succeeded in transplanting the brain by itself from one dog to the carotid–jugular vasculature in the neck of a large second dog; these isolated transplanted brains maintained their viability for periods of 6 hours to 2 days, as evidenced by the persistence of significant electrocortical activity (White, Albin, Locke, & Davidson, 1965). The significance of this research was that it showed that brain tissue en masse could be transferred surgically and survive. Basically the 1960s studies utilized host dog bodies to provide a circulatory system for adequate blood flow to the transplanted heads and brains of donor dogs. In the process, brain tissue itself was not physically altered, unlike the neural transplants in the 1979 experiments on rats where a specific area of brain was physically separated and grafted onto another brain.

As the understanding of the brain has advanced, scientists have increased their knowledge of the particular functions performed by the many different parts and tissues of the brain. While much ground remains to be covered, there is already a considerable body of information and replicated findings at hand. It is on the basis of what has been firmly established that research is moving forward. Thus, extensive knowledge of the highly selective involvement of the substantia nigra in Parkinson's disease set the stage for brain graft experiments focused on those particular brain cells.

Of course, the further recognition that degeneration of cells of the substantia nigra is associated with a dopamine deficiency in Parkinson's disease has been the basis for pharmacologic treatment of the disorder; drugs are utilized which act to increase the availability of dopamine in the brain. With Parkinson's disease, then, there is a specific site in the brain where the lesion is found; a specific tissue is involved; a specific chemical is affected; specific functional deficits result. Though many with Parkinson's disease have been significantly helped by pharmacologic interventions based on the specific neurochemical pathology, the drugs used are not without side effects which at times can be serious. Moreover, drug treatments do not arrest the underlying pathologic process of the disorder, where over time the patient's clinical condition will eventually get worse. While a number of investigators are exploring new and more effective drugs for Parkinson's disease, others have been exploring the potential value of brain grafts to replace the damaged tissue (Azmitia & Bjorklund, 1987; Madrazo et al., 1987).

Immunologically Privileged Status of the Brain

At this point it would be important to review some of the important physiologic considerations that govern the feasibility of neural transplantation. A key factor for the success of neural transplantation is the "immunologically privileged" status of the brain. Sites where tissues can be transplanted without being readily rejected are referred to as immunologically privileged. Among such sites are the brain and the eye, where antigens are apparently not easily accessible to the immune system. Corneal transplants to the eye accordingly typically do very well.

The Special Viability of Transplanted Fetal Brain Tissue

A second major consideration has been the use of fetal brain tissue in the vast majority of reports on laboratory animals to date. Fetal tissue has been used because of the greater survival rate of its transplanted cells. Most of the neural transplantation studies have used rodents where it has been found that transplanted fetal tissue survives better than neonatal grafts which in turn are superior to adult transplants—the latter reported to do very poorly (Gash et al., 1985).

Different reasons have been proposed to explain the excellent viability of fetal tissue. One important explanation is that fetal neurons may be less vulnerable to anoxia than nerve cells from adults. Neural transplantation is certainly not an instantaneous procedure, so the fact that irreversible brain damage occurs after five to ten minutes of oxygen deprivation in adult humans makes the hypoxia factor a critical consideration. Another explanation suggests that fetal antigens are especially well tolerated by the brain's immune system; that fetal brain tissue can be successfully transplanted across species lines has lent support to this view (Gash et al., 1985).

Sources of Tissue for Brain Grafts

Some additional terminology on grafts should be defined. An *autograft* involves tissue grafted from one area to another in the body of *the same individual;* this is commonly seen with skin grafts in burn victims. A *homograft* involves tissue grafted between a donor and a recipient of *the same species.* A *heterograft* involves tissue grafted between a donor and recipient of *different species.* A *xenograft* involves tissue grafted between a donor and recipient of *widely different species.*

How Brain Grafts Age

The pioneering research of Freed et al. (1980) was guided by the goal of utilizing neural transplants to treat circumscribed brain lesions. Hence, the substantia nigra, with its relatively circumscribed and progressive degeneration in Parkinson's disease, became a logical candidate for such experimentation. Transplanted fetal substantia nigra tissue from donor rats not only survived in the recipients, but endured. The grafts were found over time to contain healthy dopamine producing neurons that had a continuing positive effect on the motor behavior of the recipient rats, partially reducing the deficits in their movements.

Follow-up studies by this same research team on the same rats came up with some additional findings of great interest to investigations on the aging brain. When the host animals that had received the grafts were eventually sacrificed, they showed various changes associated with aging—discolored fur, obesity, disease, calcifications, and accumulations of the "age pigment" lipofuscin in the brain. "Despite accumulations in the brains of host animals to a degree consistent with their age, very little lipofuscin was observed in the grafts themselves. The grafts generally did not appear to be as old as the host brains, suggesting that they aged at their own rates, independent of aging of the host" (Freed et al., 1980, p. 517). The questions and speculations that spin off from these findings are intriguing indeed, spanning from new views on brain plasticity to new interventions for brain disorders. Also, in studying the response of tissue from younger animals grafted into older ones, the researcher has a unique opportunity to observe changes over time between contiguous tissues of different ages in the same organ. This could lead to another spin-off—new insights into the aging process itself.

How Grafts to Aging Brains Perform

Other studies have been carried out with the aim of examining the functioning and appearance of neural transplants in the brains of aged animals (Gash et al., 1985). One might expect that the age of the recipient's central nervous system would have a significant effect on the response of fetal brain grafts. But as described above in the research of Freed et al. (1980), this seems not to be the case; fetal grafts appear to age at different rates than older host tissue, showing fewer age effects. Moreover, brain grafts in aged rodents generally have been found to resemble neural transplants to young adult hosts with regard to growth, morphology, and functional characteristics (Gash et al., 1985). One of these studies, which compared grafts over time in young and old hosts, found no differences in the sizes of the respective grafts nor in the morphology of the neurons within the grafts. Dendritic sprouting in both age groups also appeared to be very similar. Some studies did find increased variability in the growth of grafts in older hosts as compared to younger ones, though any variation tended to be subtle.

Brain Grafts for Alzheimer's Disease?

Given encouraging results from brain graft studies on laboratory animals with Parkinsonian symptoms, curiosity has grown about other disease states characterized by circumscribed brain lesions—especially lesions involving groups of neurons associated with specific neurotransmitter deficiencies. Alzheimer's disease, alluded to above, is such a brain disease, with specific neurochemical deficits in the cholinergic system having been identified. Moreover, a specific subcortical area of the brain, known as the nucleus basalis, appears to be affected early in the course of Alzheimer's disease; this site is exceedingly rich in neurons producing the neurotransmitter acetylcholine. Hence, speculation about the potential role of brain grafts has arisen in circles of Alzheimer's disease researchers. The pathology of Alzheimer's disease, though, appears to be more complicated than that of Parkinson's disease, as further studies have uncovered additional brain sites affected in Alzheimer victims. Alzheimer's disease was discussed in considerably greater detail in Chapters 6 and 7.

Brain Grafts for Humans

So far, the studies reviewed on grafts to the brain have involved laboratory animals only. What about the transplantation of tissue to human brains? The first clinical trials of human brain grafts were reported by a Swedish group in 1985 (Backlund et al., 1985). With human organ transplants in general, the most successful have been autografts—where a patient receives his own tissue as the transplant (e.g., skin taken from one site of a person's body and grafted to a different location). The first transplants to the human brain were also autografts, and involved two patients with Parkinson's disease.

The central chemical deficit in Parkinson's disease is dopamine depletion. It is also known that the adrenal glands, located above the kidneys, contain cells (within the adrenal medulla of both glands) that produce dopamine as an intermediary compound in the synthesis of adrenaline. Earlier studies with laboratory animals sought to find out whether or not adrenal medullary tissue transplanted from the adrenal gland to the brain of the same rat would produce dopamine and act to correct experimentally induced Parkinson's disease in the animal (Freed et al., 1981). Some measure of success was achieved in the rodents. Part of this success was attributed to plasticity of the adrenal medullary tissue; when the graft was subjected to the different physiologic milieu of the brain, it was able to function compatibly with the new site. The results have led to further speculation about whether the use of nerve growth factor might facilitate even greater plasticity and adaptation of the transplanted tissue.

The treatment design proposed for the human trials followed that from the animal experiments. A Parkinsonian patient would receive a graft of tissue from his own adrenal gland—dopamine producing cells from the adrenal medulla that would be grafted to the region of the dopamine producing, but degenerating, substantia nigra in his brain. The first two human patients were a 55-year-old man and a 46-year-old woman, both of whom had been requiring increasing medication. Some positive results were reported. The change in symptomatology in the first patient was minimal, but his clinical course which had been gradually deteriorating appeared to stabilize. The second patient experienced paranoid symptoms two weeks post-surgery, with these symptoms gradually disappearing over the next two weeks. A 6-month follow-up of the second patient, though, found her Parkinsonism slightly improved. It should be pointed out that in both cases, after surgery, it was necessary to resume medication—the surgery alone was not sufficient. The investigators in this study concluded their report wondering whether a positive drug response would prove to be a prerequisite for a successful outcome of this transplantation procedure.

A more recent report by a Mexican group of an autograft of the adrenal medulla to the brain in patients with intractable Parkinson's disease described pronounced clinically positive results (Madrazo et al., 1987). This later treatment procedure differed from the earlier one by placing the graft in direct contact with cerebrospinal fluid, where it was felt the graft had better access to required nutrients. The contact with cerebrospinal fluid "also allows the chemical substances secreted by the grafted cells to be transported to other structures in the central nervous system and thus acts as a biologic infusion pump" (p. 834). One patient, a 35-year-old man, was described as having been confined to a wheelchair; 10 months after the grafting, the patient was "capable of coming to the outpatient clinic without any assistance and of playing soccer with his 5-year-old-son" (p. 833). A second patient, 39 years old, also revealed significant improvement in motor function. The authors cautioned, though, that "our results are preliminary and further work is necessary to see whether this procedure will be applicable over the long term in other types of patients with Parkinson's disease . . . particularly those who are older" (p. 831).

Subsequently, the number of patients treated by the Mexican group increased to 18. The untimely death of one of the patients from a heart attack 43 days after surgery led to a most intriguing observation. The patient had been recovering from his Parkinsonian symptoms right up to the time of his death, but from slides of the grafted cells at autopsy examination "none of the adrenal cells appeared viable" (p. 247) (Lewin, 1987). This led other investigators to speculate whether something other than or in addition to the graft might be responsible for the recovery from symptoms. One explanation offered was that "the improvement was the result of the release of trophic factors—produced either by the graft itself or by the effect of surgery on the patient's brain—that stimulated the previously faltering nigro striatal system" (p. 247) (Lewin, 1987).

Other researchers remind us that in our present understanding of Parkinson's disease, treatment is palliative, nor curative. We do not know the cause of Parkinson's disease, nor how to cure or prevent it. Drugs relieve symptoms, but do not appear to halt the underlying pathogenesis of the disorder. Grafts, too, are being looked at as potentially alleviating symptoms, and possibly slowing the course of the illness, though the transplants themselves could certainly be affected by the disease process if the cause of the disorder were not corrected (Mann, 1985).

While brain graft experimentation is moving very fast, its researchers emphasize that this field is still at a very rudimentary level of development. Note, too, that the grafts for the patients with Parkinsonism above were not transplants of brain tissue to brain tissue, but rather of adrenal tissue to brain tissue. There is a considerable amount of additional knowledge that must be gathered before transplantation of neural tissue to human brains can become a practical, appropriate clinical option (Kordower, Dean, White, & Marciano, 1988). Safety and efficacy, both on a long-term basis, need to be better understood (Sladek & Shoulson, 1988). And, there is the issue of ethics.

The need for fetal brain tissue from the donor became a major problem from the start in achieving viable neural transplants for humans, since animal studies demonstrated that brain tissue grafts from even slightly older neonates encountered difficulty taking. In using fetal homografts in humans, however, one is confronted with both ethical considerations and the practical problems of how and where to obtain human fetal tissue to graft; intense deliberations have developed in regard to both (Lewin, 1987).

Neural Transplantation and Genetic Engineering

Despite problems and the rudimentary stage of brain graft research, ideas are escalating. Bold new hypotheses are being generated, such as the potential application of recombinant DNA techniques (genetic engineering) combined with neural transplantation procedures—a marriage, so to speak, of two major frontiers of scientific investigation (Finch, 1985b). Genetically engineered cells are considered a possibility, developed via the use of recombinant DNA techniques to modify cultured cells for transplantation. Cultured neurons, it is suggested, could be manipulated so as to acquire specific DNA sequences. In turn, these DNA sequences could encode enzymes for the synthesis of specific neurotransmitters, thereby reducing chemical deficits caused by certain disorders; or perhaps they could better guide the way in which neuronal processes connect with other cells in the brain so as to improve the efficiency of cerebral functioning. Yet other ideas draw upon additional areas of scientific innovation, as with impressive new computer technologies being applied to electronic protheses.

Microchips as Brain Grafts

Medicine has moved relatively rapidly in the area of artificial implants and electronic prostheses to different parts of the body. Cardiac pacemakers and hearing aids stand out. The capacity for microcircuitry has gradually been making its way deeper and deeper within the skull. Experimental approaches to improving hearing have moved from the outer to the inner ear, while efforts to restore vision have brought technology all the way to the visual cortex of the brain. At the same time, groups of scientists are exploring the possible use of microchips to compensate for areas of damaged neurons in different parts of the brain (Freed et al., 1985). Researchers hope that such devices could potentially serve as mechanical bridges to reconnect neuronal pathways severed by pathological processes, and that they could conceivably improve the efficiency of communication among brain cells in areas altered by degenerative disease states.

A TRANSITION IN RESEARCH AND UNDERSTANDING

Historically, a very long period of time passed before scientists and society were able to recognize differences between diseases in later life and normal concomitants of the aging process (see especially Chapter 5). While this differentiation is becoming better understood, a large degree of unawareness remains about the body's remarkable capacity for resiliency in compensating for adverse changes and about the potential for repair, that continue along with aging. Certain findings significantly expand or challenge our perspective in this area. For example, a study of deer mice found that wound repair was more rapid in the *aged* mice as compared to younger ones; cutaneous wounds made on the backs of the mice healed within 3 to 4 days in the older deer mice versus 5 to 7.7 days in mature as well as young deer mice (Cohen, Cutler, & Roth, 1987). With such new findings in the field of aging research as a backdrop, the new findings in the field of brain research become all the more intriguing. Neither the "brain" nor "aging" negates capacities for resiliency or repair. The ability of the aging brain to display plasticity, and the possibility that this plasticity can be externally enhanced, brings us to the threshold of one of the most exciting new frontiers in the history of medicine and science.

9

The Aging Brain and Creativity

An examination of the aging brain would not be complete without attention to the occurrence and manifestations of creativity in later life. That the potential for creative accomplishments knows no temporal boundaries becomes apparent upon reviewing the history of human endeavor and achievement (Butler, 1967; Dennis, 1966; Lehman, 1953). Advancing chronology need not remove the potential for creative expression. Indeed, aging may be accompanied by both new opportunities as well as new forms of creative activity (McLeish, 1981; Taylor, 1974).

Examples of creativity in later life abound. While it is easier to illustrate this by looking at the well-known, they merely punctuate the point. Picasso remained prolific as a painter until he died in his 90s (from March through October in his 86th year he created 347 engravings); Verdi composed his opera *Falstaff* at age 80; Freud wrote *The Ego and the Id* at age 67; Edison was still inventing up to his death in his 80s (his last years were devoted to efforts to develop rubber latex from domestic weeds); Benjamin Franklin achieved heroic stature internationally as a diplomat in his 70s; Eubie Blake, the outstandingly talented pianist and composer of ragtime music and show tunes, continued to be in great demand as a performer well into his 90s, giving his last concert one week before his 99th birthday and receiving the Medal of Freedom earlier that year; Grandma Moses who lived to 101 turned to painting at the age of 78 when arthritis prevented her from continuing with needlework (by age 79, she had had 15 one-person shows throughout the United States and Europe); the list goes on, as does the variation in the way creativity is expressed among older adults.

WHAT IS CREATIVITY?

"Creativity" has not been an easy concept to define (Gardner, 1983). The *Britannica* (1985b) defines creativity as "the ability to make or otherwise bring into existence something new, whether a new solution to a problem, a new method or device, or a new artistic object or form." Hence, the nature of what is new or innovative can vary enormously. Not only a new theme, but a variation on that theme can be creative; so, too, can be different approaches to expressing that theme. Not surprisingly, the famous are easier to cite as examples of creative achievement in later life. But many an act of "ordinary" older individuals could well fit the *Britannica's* criteria for creativity. The remarkable adjustments and "new" strategies adopted by so many older widows following the deaths of their spouses supports this conclusion.

Different Forms and Manifestations of Creativity

The Theory of "Multiple Intelligences." Many speak of creativity as reflecting a special intelligence. Here, too, we confront complexity, as when Howard Gardner argues that "there is persuasive evidence for the existence of several *relatively autonomous* human competences," which he refers to as "human intelligences" (Gardner, 1983, p. 8). Gardner describes six such intelligences, in his theory of "Multiple Intelligences": "linguistic intelligence, musical intelligence, logical-mathematical intelligence, spatial intelligence, bodily-kinesthetic intelligence, and the personal intelligences." He then indicates:

> . . . it is appropriate to question whether personal intelligences—knowledge of self and others—should be conceived of as being at the same level of specificity (and generality) as the other intelligences . . . Perhaps it makes more sense to think of knowledge of self and others as being at a higher level, a more integrated form of intelligence, one more at the behest of the culture and of historical factors, one more truly emergent, one that ultimately comes to control and to regulate more 'primary orders' of intelligence. (p. 274)

Gardner (1983) discusses the views of the British psychologist N.K. Humphrey in emphasizing how knowledge of the social world involves creative capacities. Of Humphrey he asserts:

> In fact, he makes the bold claim that the chief creative use of human intellect lies not in the traditional areas of art and science but rather in holding society together. He points out that social primates are required to be calculating beings, to take into account the consequences of their own behavior, to calculate the

likely behavior of others, to calculate benefits and losses—all in a context where the relevant evidence is ephemeral, likely to change, even as a consequence of their own actions. Only an organism with highly developed cognitive skills can make do in such a context. The requisite abilities have been worked out over the millennia by human beings and passed on with great care and skill from the elder to the younger individuals. (p. 257)

The creative situation of the "elder" is discussed not only in terms of transferring personal knowledge to younger individuals, but from a developmental perspective where with aging one might acquire more fully developed personal knowledge. Gardner (1983) describes how various researchers in looking at the aging process and the movement to old age:

. . . stress processes of continued development, where an individual has the option of becoming increasingly autonomous, integrated, or self-actualized, provided that he can make the correct "moves" and arrive at a suitable stance of accepting what cannot be altered. The end-goal of these developing processes is a self that is highly developed and fully differentiated from others: desirable models would include Socrates, Jesus Christ, Mahatma Gandhi, Eleanor Roosevelt—individuals who appear to have understood much about themselves and about their societies and to have come to terms successfully with the frailties of the human condition, while at the same time inspiring others around them to lead more productive lives. (p. 252)

Three of Gardner's four examples are of individuals who clearly achieved new creative heights in later life, the fourth not having had the opportunity to live that long. The force of Socrates' ideas at 71 years of age was such that his convictions provoked a State trial that resulted in his death sentence and nearly 25 centuries of philosophical debate over his final views; with Mahatma Gandhi, the force of his later life presence was well reflected through his culminating influence in negotiating for an autonomous Indian state at the age of 77; in the case of Eleanor Roosevelt, the force of circumstances and her personality moved her from a housewife in her youth to a humanitarian of the world in her seventh decade, when she served as chairman of the United Nations Commission on Human Rights.

The Concept of the "Ulyssean Adult."   In leading up to his definition of creativity, McLeish discusses the views of Abraham Maslow on creativity. Maslow separated creativity into two types—"special talent creativity" and "self-actualizing creativeness" (Maslow, 1959). McLeish (1981) elaborates:

First, "special talent creativity"—the creativity of the gifted inventor, scientist, poet, sculptor, architect, novelist, and so on; and second, "self-actualizing creativeness," which Maslow defined as showing itself much more in creative changes in the personality, and in a tendency to do anything creatively—that is *living* creatively. (p. 96)

Interestingly, aspects of Howard Gardner's theory of "personal intelligences" bear some resemblance to Maslow's concept of "self-actualizing creativeness."

McLeish (1981) then offers his own definition of creativity,

. . . the process by which a person employs both conscious and unconscious domains of the mind to combine various existing materials into fresh constructions or configurations that, in some degree, cause significant changes in the self-system of the person concerned, or significantly alter the environment surrounding the person, whether such a change is great or small. (p. 96)

McLeish addresses the essence of this definition and the concept of "self-actualization" in his own concept of the "Ulyssean Adult" which he feels personifies the potential for continuing creativity in one's later years. He was influenced by the portrayal of Ulysses in Tennyson's poem that drew upon Homer's depiction of the same mythical hero 2600 years earlier in *The Odyssey*. Tennyson's aging Ulysses invites,

> "Come my friends,
> "Tis not too late to seek a newer world.
> Push off, and sitting well in order smite
> The surrounding furrows; for my purpose holds
> To sail beyond the sunset, and the baths
> Of all the western stars, until I die.
> It may be that the gulfs will wash us down:
> It may be we shall touch the Happy Isles,
> And see the great Achilles, whom we knew.
> Tho' much is taken, much abides; and tho'
> We are not now that strength which in old days
> Moved earth and heaven; that which we are, we are;
> One equal temper of heroic hearts,
> Made weak by time and fate, but strong in will
> To strive, to seek, to find, and not to yield."

McLeish (1976) then attempts to portray those qualities which especially identify the Ulyssean person in later life:

When, therefore, in our own time we see a man or woman in the later years who maintains the questing spirit, and who does so with courage and resourcefulness in a wide variety of circumstances, many of them terribly, even tragically adverse, such a man or woman may well be described as Ulyssean. The quest, the courage, and the resourcefulness may be exhibited on a human stage of immense proportions or in total solitariness and obscurity. It is not the time or the location but the quality of the life being lived that creates the Ulyssean Adult. (p. 13)

As but one example, McLeish then goes on to list 125 noted scientists from all fields "who were incontestably richly creative into their late, even very late years" (McLeish, 1976, p. 287); these names were obtained from a small but thorough review he made in 1975. Such achievement is certainly not unique to scientists, as illustrated by the Supreme Court Justices in the United States. Among the first 15 Chief Supreme Court Justices from John Jay (appointed by Washington) to Warren Burger (retiring under Reagan), 11 were 65 or older while serving; and 10 (fully *two-thirds*) were over 70 while sitting as Chief Justices.

Other "Patterns" of Creativity. Taylor has postulated five "behavioral dispositions" toward creativity, which essentially follow a developmental sequence—the fifth disposition emerging with greatest strength in later life (Taylor, 1974): (1) "expressive spontaneity" is described as the earliest form, appearing, for example, in the spontaneous drawings or extemporaneous dance of children; (2) "technical proficiency" is portrayed as the next form, reflected in specific skills that are developed as adolescence is approached; (3) "inventive ingenuity" comes next, which Taylor suggests is apparent in idealized drawings or the use of gadgetry often seen in adolescence and the early 20s; (4) "innovative flexibility" is depicted as emerging in the late 20s to late 30s, where basic ideas are adapted for new purposes; (5) "emergentive originality" is what Taylor calls the capacity to create original or essentially new ideas, a disposition he views as "flourishing in the late 50s and 60s, indeed for many people into their 80s and 90s."

STUDIES OF CREATIVITY IN LATER LIFE

Studies of Performance, Achievement, and Productivity with Aging

Researchers have tended to study creativity among older adults in terms of achievement, performance, productivity, and creative expression. Moreover, they have looked at such accomplishment in the face of long-held beliefs that creativity and achievement are adversely affected by age per se. Certainly McLeish's study above of 125 noted scientists whose creative accomplishments remained robust well into their later years challenges such popular views.

Cole compared the work published by scientists from six different fields of inquiry—scientists from under age 35 to those over 60 (Cole,

1979). His study was particularly important, since it distinguished longitudinal research findings from cross-sectional ones. Cross-sectional investigations, as pointed out earlier, compare different individuals from different cohort groups (different generations); longitudinal research offers a far better assessment of the age factor, since it focuses on the same individuals as they themselves age. Cole also attempted in an interesting way to separate qualitative considerations from quantitative ones. In other words, he tried to focus on the quality of a paper published by a scientist in earlier adulthood as compared to one published in later adulthood. This was done by determining the number of citations each paper received, regarding citations as a reflection of how the general community of scientists valued any particular paper.

Cole's cross-sectional results are tabulated in Table 9.1. From the table it is apparent even from cross-sectional data that the creative productivity of scientists can be maintained at a significant level as they age. Moreover, Cole points out that there are important factors other than age per se that can account for certain ostensible fall-offs with aging. For example, illness would cut down on the capacity of creative persons to continue performing at the same level, while death would reduce the number of creative individuals. Moreover, every area of creative endeavor has its own reward system which influences creative behavior independent of the age factor. Thus, in science, Cole (1979) hypothesizes that "those who are not rewarded are less likely to continue publishing. Thus, as a cohort of scientists advance in age the number of prolific publishers is likely to decline. Most people will not continue an activity as arduous as scientific research unless they are rewarded for it." Those "who continue to publish throughout their careers are a 'residuc' composed of the best members of their cohort" (p. 969). Put differently, the brightest lights in many fields are often capable of burning strong throughout the life cycle. Of course, not all creative individuals

Table 9.1 Age and Average
Number of Citations to Work Published
During 1965–1969 by Scientists in Six Fields [a]

Age of scientists	Av. no. citations in chemistry, geology, mathematics physics, psychology, and sociology
Under 35	7.5
35–39	8.8
40–44	9.1
45–49	6.4
50–59	5.7
60+	6.3

[a] Adapted from Cole (1979).

receive their just rewards. This could explain why "over time" (as opposed to resulting from advancing age), creative accomplishments may seem to fall off. The fall-off may reflect lack of reward over time rather than lack of capacity for creative expression in later life.

Cole's longitudinal data are even more striking. He reviewed the work of a given group of mathmaticians over a 25-year period following their receiving their Ph.D.'s. Here he found that both the quantity and the quality of their papers remained constant (see Table 9.2). Cole's conclusion is succinctly stated: "The long-standing belief that age is negatively associated with scientific productivity and creativity is shown to be based upon incorrect analysis of the data" (p. 958).

It should also be recognized that older scientists often reroute creative energies. They commonly take on administration and teaching duties, cutting down on basic research.

Other investigators have similarly carried out studies suggesting that significant intellectual and creative achievement is "more or less continuous over the whole life span (Alpaugh, Parham, Cole, & Birren, 1982; Bullough, Bullough, & Mauro, 1978; Maduro, 1974; Torrance, 1977). What is more, Bullough and colleagues (1978) see in their research findings "an implication that achievement is related to the ability to survive"—that those with greater longevity have had more opportunity to bring their work to greater fruition and maturity. As for those who believe that original and creative inspiration is more likely to take place before age 40, Bullough and colleagues propose that such originality and inspiration is usually not recognized unless followed by continual repetition, retesting, refinement, or evolution. To test their hypothesis about the positive correlation between creativity and longevity, these researchers studied intellectual and creative achievers in two historical periods "of significant intellectual and creative achievement—18th-century Scotland and 15th-century Florence." The 15th century, of

Table 9.2 Average Number of Papers Published and Citations to Them for a Specific Group of Mathematicians Receiving Ph.D.'s from 1947 to 1950[a]

Date of publication	Av. no. papers published	Av. no. citations listed
1950–1954	2.4	0.84
1955–1959	2.8	1.2
1960–1964	2.3	1.1
1965–1969	2.8	1.4
1970–1974	2.6	1.1

[a]Adapted from Cole (1979).

course, was known as the *Renaissance,* and the 18th century the *Enlightenment* (or the *Age of Reason*).

Age at death was examined among 375 eminent 18th-century Scottish achievers and 158 eminent 15th-century Florentine achievers. The significance of age becomes more apparent upon considering census data. In 18th-century Scotland, the median age of death of those in the general population who survived their first year was around 40; the median age of death among the Scottish achievers, however, was over 70, with 21% of the achiever group living beyond 80 years of age. For 15th-century Florence, there are no comparable census data. But for those in the general population who survived their 21st birthday, death came on the average a decade earlier than in 18th-century Scotland; the median age of death among the Florentine achievers, though, was 61, with 31% of the achiever group living beyond 70 years of age. Hence, increased age— particularly having lived to over age 60 during the Renaissance in 15th-century Florence and over the age of 70 during the Enlightenment in 18th-century Scotland—has been found to be closely associated with increased eminence in intellectual and creative achievement.

The noted historian Arnold Toynbee saw the advantage of increased age in a similar light. Writing at the age of 77 Toynbee (1969) offered that:

> Every stage of life has its own ordeals and own rewards. My reward for having reached my present age is that this has given me time to carry out more than the whole of my original agenda; and an historian's work is of the kind in which time is a necessary condition for achievement. (p. 124)

The Search for Connections Between Human Development and Creativity in Later Life

Students of gerontology have long wondered whether there are unique developmental patterns, tendencies, or potentials in later life. Taylor's concept of "emergentive originality," described above, represents one such postulate. Maduro (1974) adds cross-cultural perspective from his research on elderly folk painters in India:

> With increasing years creative artists say they are "more open" to the nuances of internal chaos and pure intuition, to "conceiving," and to "the unfolding of the self" than to reinforcing the ascendency of the ego's executive functions over the entire psychic apparatus. It is as if ego is expected to give up control from the top down for the rewards of a more wholeness-fostering dialogue with creative unconscious processes. (p. 308)

From a related perspective the psychoanalyst Grotjahn (1955) wrote about resistance to psychologically charged issues being weakened in later life, associating this development with a new potential for insight or expression (see discussion of psychotherapy and aging in Chapter 5). Certainly, Mark Twain would have found no fault with this observation, characteristically commenting in an essay he wrote on his 70th birthday (Twain, 1963):

> The seventieth birthday! It is the time of life when you arrive at a new and awful dignity; when you may throw aside the decent reserves which have oppressed you for a generation and stand unafraid and unabashed upon your seven-terraced summit and look down and teach—unrebuked. (p. 469)

The teaching that Twain referred to has long been regarded a major creative contribution of elder members of societies. Much attention has been focused on the great debt owed to the elderly or old for their essential role in preserving wisdom that slowly accrued in primitive societies. Simmons (1945) reflected:

> Among preliterate peoples, memories have been the only repositories of knowledge, skills, and rituals. Where writing and records have been unknown— where all that was worth knowing had to be carried in the head—a lucid mind, a good memory, and a seasoned judgment, even housed in a feeble frame, have been indispensable and treasured assets to the group. Those endowed with the art of writing and surrounded by printed documents can scarcely appreciate the inestimable value of an aged person possessing more knowledge than any other source within reach. There are unlimited examples of the role of the aged as custodians of folk wisdom. (p. 131)

Butler (1967) has attempted to list certain capacities and potential functions in society associated with middle and later life, including: accumulated knowledge and skills, philosophical development, judgment, wisdom, counseling, teaching, candor, honesty, empathy, serenity, dependability, and prestige. The application of these capacities or functions can obviously permit different forms of creative behavior.

Indeed, concepts of creative capacity deriving from a uniqueness of one's later years are not new. In his nearly two-thousand-year-old writings *On Old Age,* Lucius Annaeus Seneca stressed that "the apples are never so good than when they begin to wither and ripen" (Seneca, 1926, p. 46). Seneca himself wrote some of his best philosophical works upon his retirement in his seventh decade.

Creativity in Response to Loss in Later Life.

In ancient Greek mythology, Tiresias was a Theban who had the misfortune of observing the goddess Athena while she was undressing to bathe. Outraged, Athena blinded Tiresias. But Zeus took pity upon the poor mortal, and replaced Tiresias' loss of outer vision with great insight and prophetic powers that both grew with aging and facilitated long life for the seer. One is reminded of the poet and physician William Carlos Williams who, following a stroke in his sixties, turned full time to his verse, writing about "an old age that adds as it takes away" (Foy, 1979). Williams was posthumously awarded the Pulitzer Prize in poetry for his *Pictures from Brueghel and Other Poems,* published at age 79, the year before he died. The myth of Tiresias and the mastery of William Carlos Williams point out the very real potential for creativity in response to loss in later life.

Leon Edel (1979), in studying artists as they age, looked at the rage of William Butler Yeats in the poet's later years. Edel saw Yeats as manifesting a "controlled rage"—in part a response to his perceived "loss" of youth. "Yeats flamed and the flames were brighter for his being old. He had never flamed as much in his youth" (p. 212). Edel elaborated:

> When he went to Stockholm to receive the Nobel Prize, Yeats looked at the medal that came to him with Sweden's bounty; it showed a young man listening to the Muse. Yeats thought: "I was good-looking once like that young man, but my unpracticed verse was full of infirmity, my Muse old as it were; and now I am old and rheumatic, and nothing to look at, but my Muse is young. I am even persuaded that she is like those Angels in Swedenborg's vision, and moves perpetually 'towards the day-spring of her youth.'" Let us remind ourselves that when the Angels of Swedenborg kissed, the kiss was a burst of flame. (p. 211)

The playwright Sean O'Casey at age 77 reviewed his past, present, and future in terms of creative performance and potential, in the process providing further illustrations of new creative expression following loss in later life (O'Casey, 1968):

> Does creativity decline with age? No. Activity is bound to be less, but the creativity of an active mind goes on . . . even in the face of age's infirmities, difficulties can be conquered by the determined will . . . . Beethoven wrote his greatest symphony when he was deaf; Prescott wrote his monumental work on *The Conquest of Mexico* when he was half-blind; and Renoir painted on when he had to tie a brush to a rheumatic hand . . . . In a few months . . . I shall be seventy-eight . . . . I have just finished a new play; I am working on a new book; I write many letters, and here, now, I am telling those who may be a little younger, or as old as myself, to go on too. (p. 953)

Grandma Moses provides yet another illustration—at two levels—of the capacity to mobilize creativity in response to loss: Following the death of her husband, she began to embroider pictures; with the later loss of agility in manipulating a needle, Grandma Moses began to paint and achieved fame.

Returning to the earlier point about widows, the concomitance of loss and creative adaptation can again be observed. Certain well-known widows highlight the phenomenon for those lacking fame but not accomplishment. The image of Eleanor Roosevelt has provided a mirror for many women losing a spouse in their later years. Although already accomplished, Eleanor Roosevelt rose to even greater heights in the midst of bouts of loneliness in her widowhood. President Truman appointed her a delegate to the United Nations, where she served during her sixties and seventies, playing a major role in the drafting and adoption of the Universal Declaration of Human Rights. Her many travels across the globe and meetings with most of the leaders of the world around critical social and humanitarian issues made her legend. Her autobiography *On My Own,* written at age 74, appropriately begins with the opening chapter "An End and a Beginning." In it she wrote (Roosevelt, 1958):

> In the years since 1945 (the death of Franklin Delano Roosevelt) I have known the various phases of loneliness that are bound to occur when people no longer have a busy family life. But, without particularly planning it, I have made the necessary adjustments to a different way of living, and I have enjoyed almost every minute of it and almost everything about it. (p. 2)

A Changing Creativity with Aging.   While there are those who experience a decline in creativity with aging, there are others whose particular form of creative expression continues throughout the life cycle (Alpaugh, Parham, Cole, & Birren, 1982; Cole, 1979; Hearn, 1972). There are those for whom later life provides a time for further development, ultimate refinement, or even full flowering of their lifelong work (Edel, 1979; Maduro, 1974). For others, the nature of their creativity may vary as they age, with different manifestations of the creative process at different stages of their lives (Lieberman & Lieberman, 1983). James Hutton, an 18th-century Scotsman, fits the last group. Hutton no doubt was counted among the eminent Scottish achievers during the period of the Enlightenment in the above study (Bullough et al., 1978) on the relationship of longevity to achievement.

As a young man Hutton developed an interest in chemistry, but as he added years entered the legal profession, subsequently moving into medicine where he acquired an M.D. degree. From medicine Hutton went on to devote himself to agriculture, and eventually to geology where in his seventh decade his extraordinary theories and discoveries led to him being referred to as "the founder of modern geology" (Bailey, 1967). His historic findings and observations are contained in his major two-volume work,

Theory of the Earth, which he published in 1795 as he approached his seventieth birthday. Among other things, Hutton's contributions to geology have helped in the better understanding of how the earth "ages."

Hutton was the originator of one of the most fundamental principles of geology—uniformitarianism (*Britannica,* 1985f). Basically, uniformitarianism is a doctrine that explains the formation, features, and aging of the earth's surface in natural terms. The doctrine was revolutionary in two different ways. It not only challenged existing geological theory but it provoked extreme reactions in theological thinking as well. Up until Hutton's theory, the prevailing view was that the earth and its crust had formed through supernatural means some 6,000 years earlier, shaped by such catastrophic events as the Great Flood described in the Bible. Hutton showed how the earth was much older, how soils were formed by the weathering of rocks, and how layers of sediment accumulated.

The effect of Hutton's ideas on the learned world at that time has been compared with the earlier revolution in thought brought about by Copernicus (16th century) and Galileo (17th century) whose observations, theories, and experiments showed how the earth revolved around the sun, not the other way around; this suggested both scientifically and philosophically that the earth was not the center of the universe or of creation as had been the thrust of Biblical teachings. Understandably, these concepts unleashed a storm of criticism.

It is of note that, prior to its publication, the finished copy of Copernicus' classic work *The Revolutions of the Celestial Spheres* was only brought to Copernicus on the last day of his life at the age of 70. Of similar note is that Galileo's monumental work *Dialogue Concerning Two New Sciences* was completed when the scientist was 70 years old; this work, which recapitulated the results of Galileo's early experiments and included his mature thoughts on the principles of mechanics, has been considered his most valuable publication. Due to the religious uproar resulting from Galileo's experiments and lectures that upheld Copernican doctrine, Galileo was placed under house arrest for the final eight years of his life until his death at the age of 77.

The 18th-century views of Hutton came under related attack. It was this attack, though, that pushed Hutton to fully develop his ideas and conclusions and to publish them in his master work completed at the end of his seventh decade. Utilizing Huttonian principles, Sir Charles Lyell, another celebrated Scottish geologist, published his classic work *Principles of Geology.* Lyell's work, in turn, profoundly influenced Charles Darwin who in 1859 published his revolutionary treatise *On the Origin of Species by Means of Natural Selection.* Darwin's writings on evolution in effect applied to animals and plants the theory of uniformitarianism that Hutton had developed about earth.

Again, one need look not only to the well known to witness phenomena such as changing creative expression with aging. A study of 70 persons between 50 and 87 years of age who developed second careers as artists or craftspersons offers further illustration and perspective on such change (Lieberman & Lieberman, 1983); in each case, the new direction in art represented a significant departure from earlier areas of involvement such as business, law, and engineering.

A STUDY OF CREATIVITY AMONG CENTENARIANS

As already emphasized, creativity in later life is not confined to the famous. Perhaps this point is best made by looking at a remarkable study of centenarians—100-year-olds who show that it is not just a Grandma Moses who can shine with advanced age, and that Grandma Moses was not the only centenarian who ever stood out. When Victor Christgau was Executive Director of the Social Security Administration, district offices of that agency across the country interviewed social security recipients who were at least 100 years old or within only a few months of that age. Structured interviews with 1,132 centenarians were carried out and published by the Social Security Administration during 1963–1972 in 13 now-rare softbound volumes. Cutler (1978) subsequently published a book based on those interviews. Some citations from that book follow:

A visit to centenarian Robert Adger Bowen in Greenville, South Carolina, was not a trip through a time machine. In spite of his 100 years, he seemed very much a citizen of these times. One had only to turn to the editorial page of *The Greenville News* to see his letters on every issue of the day . . . . Another of Mr. Bowen's interests was the Foundation for Historic Restoration in the Pendleton Area. This organization was restoring Ashabula, one of his mother's homes. Mr. Bowen had recently compiled two books of his poetry: *When Sweet Birds Sing* and *Footfalls and Echoes,* whose profit went into the foundation. (p. 22)

Mrs. Bainbridge (of Hollywood, California), an avid reader, said she read the *Los Angeles Times* from cover to cover each day . . . . She still continued to work in the song-writing field. This was her major interest or hobby, aside from her continued interest in Christian Science. She had several songs published in 1961 (two years earlier) and had others being considered for publication. (p. 25)

Some centenarians create with no apparent thought of an audience. For them, the act of self-expression is reward enough in itself. So it was with Moses G. Weaver of Salt Lake City . . . . Mr. Weaver (who worked at 43 different jobs during his life, from farming to watchmaking) said he had been writing poetry since he was 16 years old. He had a loose-leaf binder full of his poems. They were well-written and showed a keen insight into human life and accomplishments . . . . He also enjoyed pencil drawings and had a large number of beautiful ones completed during the past decade. They showed close attention to minute details such as facial expressions. (p. 27)

George W. Beynon (of St. Petersburg, Florida), upon retirement as a bridge official, organized a new venture. Although over 90, he started a unique correspondence school for bridge-tournament directors. At the time of his hundredth-birthday interview, he still played the piano, drove his car to bridge tournaments, and startled the unwary with his vigorous handshake. His school had more than 800 students. On the side, he wrote a bridge column for the *St. Petersburg Times.* (p. 36)

Centenarian Helen Hasse of Tyron, North Carolina, when asked if she had any outside activities responded, "I have over 50 correspondents. I write a good many letters. I also make up rhymes. I have had some published in the *Chicago Tribune.* Some of my letters I type myself, and some I write longhand. Also, I make infant garments and little blankets and send them to the welfare department and the health department to be given to needy mothers for their children, and that takes all the money I have over my regular expenses. I have many friends who send me gifts of money, and it all goes for this material. I estimate that I have made by hand over 2,000 garments in the past several years, and all of them have been distributed to the needy." (p. 79)

Other reports similarly document the potential for creative capacity even in those who reach 100 years of age (de Beauvoir, 1978; Palmore, 1987; Segerberg, 1982).

WHAT ABOUT PHYSICAL CAPACITY IN CREATIVE ACTS WITH AGING?

As the facts are examined and the stereotypes retired, the creative potential that resides in the aging mind becomes more apparent. Less apparent but still real is the robustness or resiliency that can remain with the aging body to complement the capacity of the aging brain (Finch & Schneider, 1985). We can perhaps appreciate this more readily when looking at aging artists and musicians who combine creativity in their imagery or compositions with physical dexterity in beautifully executing their works. A long list could be given, from Pablo Picasso to Pablo Cassals—the former remaining so magnificently adept on the canvas, the latter on the cello. To push the point, consider the remarkable achievement of Sir Francis Chichester, described in his autobiography *Gypsy Moth Circles the World* which he wrote at the age of 65 (Chichester, 1968). Chichester, at the age of 65, carried out a dream that demanded the fortitude of both the mind and the body—a physical challenge never before accomplished by another at any age. At 65 years of age, Sir Francis C. Chichester sailed round the world, *alone.*

On August 27, 1966 Chichester began a solo sail around the world in his 54 foot boat, the *Gypsy Moth.* He had his 65th birthday at sea on September 17, 1966, and completed his circumnavigation of the globe on May 28, 1967. In the process, he established seven world records at that time, including the fastest voyage circling the earth by any small sailing vessel (approximately twice as fast as any other) and the longest passage that had been made by such a vessel before making a port call. Chichester wrote in his log:

> People keep at me about my age. I suppose they think that I can beat age. I am not that foolish. Nobody, I am sure can be more aware than I am that my time is limited. I don't think I can escape aging, but why beef about it? Our only purpose in life, if we are able to say such a thing, is to put up the best performance we can—in anything, and only in so doing lies satisfaction in living.

Hemingway, in 1952, wrote *The Old Man and the Sea,* a short but poignant novel that played a part in his gaining the Nobel Prize for Literature in 1954 (Hemingway, 1980). The author mixed trial, tragedy, and ultimately triumph in describing the relentless, agonizing battle of an old fisherman, alone at sea with only a skiff, battling a giant marlin and a group of sharks. The story portrays the struggle, courage, and quest for mastery and fulfillment of a dream that know no endpoint in the life cycle. About the old man, Hemingway wrote: "Everything about him was old except his eyes and they were the same color as the sea and were cheerful and undefeated . . . man is not made for defeat . . . . A man can be destroyed but not defeated" (p. 103).

Writing about Sir Francis Chichester, a colleague described Chichester as "at last releasing the dream." In so doing, Chichester was knighted by the Queen with the very sword given by Queen Elizabeth I to Sir Francis Drake upon his voyage around the world by sail nearly four centuries earlier. Though Magellan's crew (1519–1522) was the first to sail around the world earlier in the 16th century, Magellan himself was killed on route. Drake later circled the earth by ship (1577–1580) and lived to tell about it. Drake had a crew; Chichester had none. Chichester's colleague wrote (Anderson, 1968):

> Chichester cannot write this epilogue, because he could not see himself as the crowd of cheering Londoners saw him. I did. Slight (until you caught a glimpse of the muscle in wrist and forearm), weatherbeaten, wearing thick glasses, Chichester gave himself no airs, and when he acknowledged the Lord Mayor's

address of welcome, the crowd's cheers, he spoke more of Sheila his wife and Giles his son than of himself. He was the nation's hero, but to me he seemed to epitomize not scarlet and lace, but that incredible endurance that the people of England have shown when it was needed of them, the endurance of men who sailed with Drake, Anson, Cook and Nelson, for England. And that, I think, is what everybody felt. And that is why we cheered. (p. 223)

Such cheering about the likes of Chichester, Hutton, and the lot of older persons keeping the creative process alive across the life cycle would have been easily understood by the great 19th-century American poet Walt Whitman who published up until he died in his eighth decade. About old age, he wrote in his celebrated work *Leaves of Grass:*

> Youth, large, lusty, loving—
>   youth, full of grace, force, fascination,
> Do you know that Old Age may come after you,
>   with equal grace, force, fascination?

Equally we might speculate on the questions of *why* the brain and the body as a whole age and *what,* if anything, we can do about it. That is the focus of the next and final chapter of this book.

10

Theories of Aging and Life Extension

The aging of the brain needs to be looked at within the context of theories of aging in general (Bailey, 1987; Birren & Bengtson, 1988; Warner, Butler, Sprott, & Schneider, 1987). Be they plant or animal, all living things are generally believed to age in species-specific patterns (Hayflick, 1987a; Hendricks & Hendricks, 1977). But there are animals where aging has yet to be demonstrated (Comfort, 1979); there are some fish and amphibians that have an indeterminate life-span, leaving the universality of aging unproven (Hayflick, 1987a). Indeterminate life-span, though, is not the equivalent of immortality, since organisms eventually die of disease, accidents, or other environmental factors at a rate apart from the aging process.

Life-spans are as brief as 24 hours in the common mayfly to as long as 12,000 to 15,000 years with the *Macrozamia* tree which grows in the Tambourine Mountains of Queensland, Australia (Kendig & Hutton, 1979; Rockstein, Chesky, & Sussman, 1977). Among animals, longevity records point to tortoises with documentation around the 170-year mark for the oldest. The female of any one species generally outlives the male, though there are exceptions among mammals; the stallion has a greater life-span than the mare, while the male Syrian hamster lives longer than the female (Rockstein, Chesky, & Sussman, 1977). The reports of long-livers among humans have turned out to be grossly misleading (Busse & Blazer, 1980c). Media stories for years have identified groups of individuals across the globe as being well over a hundred years of age. These groups have included the *Los Viejos* (the very old) in the small Andes Mountain village of Vilcabamba in Ecuador, the Hunzukuts of the Karakoram Range in Kashmir, and the Abkhazians of the Republic of Georgia in the U.S.S.R. A series of studies was made of these various groups, and the most consistent finding was fibs (Bennett & Garson, 1986). Self-reports of very old age had been greatly exaggerated. Russian scientists also participated in the Soviet Georgia studies where the oldest resident was determined to be only 96 years of age. Where records exist and age has been substantiated, documentation shows the oldest human may have been Pierre Joubert, who was born July 15, 1701, and died November 16, 1814, aged 113 years and 124 days (*Britannica*, 1985d).

WHY DO LIVING THINGS AGE?

To ask why living things age is to ask two questions—one about purpose, the other about process: (1) What purpose does aging serve; are there advantages to aging that benefit different species and outweigh disadvantages; what would the consequences be of not aging? (2) What is the biological process of aging; how does aging happen; what are the factors that influence the nature and rate of aging?

In short, it is difficult to answer either question and the different components of each one. Major disagreements exist among researchers who have attempted different explanations (Hayflick, 1987a; Kirkwood, 1985). As to the biological (process) explanation of why aging occurs, how it is induced, and what affects its rate, over a dozen theories have been put forth; they will be reviewed below in the section, "Theories of Aging"; many of these biological theories are interesting, informative, or provocative, but ultimately none answers the basic questions unequivocally.

As to the question of purpose, researchers cannot agree as to whether it is adaptive or nonadaptive to age—greatly complicating theories as to why and how aging evolved. Two recurrent themes emerge in theories that aging is adaptive (Kirkwood, 1985): "(1) that aging is necessary to eliminate old individuals from the population to provide space and nutriment for their progeny (this is the 'living space argument'); (2) that possession of a finite life span ensures a more rapid succession of generations and thus improves the chance of a species adapting to changes in its environment" (p. 36). On the other hand, two arguments speak against "adaptive" theories of aging (Kirkwood, 1985):

(1) Accidental mortality is sufficiently high in most species that obvious senility is rarely seen in wild populations. Thus, the "living space" argument does not hold up, and there is neither need for a mechanism specifically to terminate life nor opportunity for it to evolve.

(2) For aging to have arisen as an adaptive trait would have required that its selection for advantage to the species or group was more effective than selection among individuals within the group for the reproductive advantages of a longer life. Superiority of the former kind of selection over the latter is very seldom the case. (p. 37)

Still, the view of aging as an adaptive process is widely popular. The "living space" argument above addresses biological or physical aspects of available space (e.g., whether there would be sufficient food were it not for aging); it does not consider social considerations that with humans would add to the "adaptive" argument. Adaptive aspects of aging from a psychosocial perspective are implicit in the following fairy tale (Chinen 1987, p. 341):

Once upon a time, a great king went hunting with his comrades. They stopped for lunch at the summit of a hill. The king then lamented the thought of his own death, and how he would lose everything. His nobles also bemoaned the thought of their deaths. One among them laughed, however. The king ignored the laughter and went on to wish for immortality. His lords chimed in agreement, but the last noble laughed again. The lords demanded the reason for their comrade's laughter, but he would not explain. Finally the king himself demanded the reason. The lord acquiesced, and said he was thinking about what it would be like if they all lived forever. In that case, the First King would still be alive, and the Great Sage, and all the other heroes of history. Compared to them, the King would be only a clerk, and they, only peasants! That thought made him laugh. After a tense moment, the king raised his drinking glass and penalized the other nobles two draughts of wine each for encouraging his royal vanity.

Of course, while a social argument for aging as an adaptive process may be highly relevant to man, it is another matter with mice and other species; they all age.

THEORIES OF AGING

Theories of aging include attention to factors intrinsic to the organism, on the one hand, and extrinsic to it, on the other, that influence the aging process. Intrinsic factors would include internal, inborn variables, such as genetic programming; extrinsic ones would include external elements, such as the role of stress or infection. Sometimes it is difficult to decide whether a component is intrinsic or extrinsic. Atherosclerosis is a case in point (Walton, 1978). Many have viewed atherosclerosis as going with the territory of aging, and until recently it was commonly (erroneously) thought to be the basis for senility or Alzheimer's disease (see Chapter 6).

Moreover, among entire populations of people, such as the Mali tribes in Africa and the Yemenite Jews, atherosclerotic vascular disease is typically not found (Bierman, 1985; Hendricks & Hendricks, 1977). Evidence of this nature suggests that atherosclerosis is not unequivocally an intrinsic phenomenon, or at least not an unmodifiable inherent process, but is influenced by external factors such as nutrition and/or stress. Still, when atherosclerosis becomes manifest it is often associated with various cardiac ailments that develop more often with aging.

To the extent that external factors over time bring about various diseases and disabilities associated with aging, they have been described as contributing to a "secondary aging" process (Busse, 1978). "Primary aging," accordingly, refers to changes induced by intrinsic processes. Major theories of why aging occurs will now be reviewed in greater detail; some of them have become the basis of attempts at life extension which will also be reviewed below. By the end of the discussion it will become apparent that there is no unified theory of aging, nor resolution as to wha' clearly causes the aging process. The search for life extension, it will be seen, is at a similar stage of understanding.

Entropy Theory/Exhaustion Theory/Wear and Tear Theory

One of the oldest theories of aging has been referred to in at least three different ways—as the entropy theory, or the exhaustion theory, or the wear and tear theory (Busse & Blazer, 1980c; Hayflick, 1987a). Biological and psychological theories are not uncommonly influenced by prevailing physical theories. The Second Law of Thermodynamics, formulated in the 19th century, applies here. It contends that energy becomes increasingly unavailable to do work or maintain order, a quality described as entropy. In other words, the tendency for a system to run down or to move toward disorganization due to energy loss is referred to as entropy. Like a machine with a fixed reserve of energy or a windup clock, the individual in aging was seen to experience a gradual exhaustion of capacity and efficiency over time. But there are problems with this theory. For example, regular work and exercise, which utilize considerable energy, keep the individual in tone, often increasing the interval between periods of exhaustion, and commonly make the person look the better for wear.

Cell Death Theories/the Genetic Programming or Commitment Theory

Cells die for many reasons. Trauma, diseases, radiation, toxins, and other external or environmental factors can damage or destroy human cells throughout the body. There are two groups of scientists who hypothesize that what controls the aging process is the life and death of the body's cells (Busse, 1978). One group has postulated that over time cumulative insults to cells build up to the point of causing a progressive change called aging, eventually leading to death. The second group says that were this the case, there would be much more variation in the course of aging and in the number of years one might live; instead, they suggest that much more likely is a genetically built-in limit to the life of a cell, and therefore to the life of the organism. Most organs of the body have cells that divide so as to produce new cells. It used to be thought that many of these cells could divide indefinitely, that age was irrelevant to them. Subsequent research, however, came up with the remarkable finding that there is a given number of doublings for a cell before the divisions cease (Hayflick, 1977). Why this happens is speculative. These studies have also found that cells produced late in life reveal morphological differences from the same types of cells produced by younger organisms. Additionally, after a certain period of time has passed, the rate of cell division starts to decline, eventually coming to a stop, with cell death ensuing. A further finding was that the number of doublings did not differ as a factor of the sex of the organism from which the cells were taken, suggesting that other intrinsic and/or extrinsic factors need to be explored to explain differential mortality between men and women.

From these studies it was concluded that the genesis of aging and the cause of death were genetically programmed in the cell. Genes supposedly set a biologic time clock for cells to begin to slow and then to cease divisions. Genetics would, in effect, install a memory in the cell committing it at some point to dying. This theory, too, is not without its critics, some of whom like earlier investigators think that under the proper conditions cells would be capable of continuous reduplication and not be committed to death (Holliday, Hutschtscha, Tarrant, & Kirkwood, 1977). At the same time, there is one type of cell that does appear to exhibit the capacity for immortality—the cancer cell (Hayflick, 1987b). Curiously, the frequency of cancer cells increases with aging.

The Genetic Mutation Theory/the Error Theory

The genetic mutation or genetic error theories reflect a combination of extrinsic and intrinsic factor considerations (Busse, 1978). Extrinsic factors are hypothesized to alter the actions of intrinsic factors such that aging is the outcome. Since DNA is the genetic brain of a cell—telling it what to do, what proteins to synthesize—a radiation-induced mutation in the DNA could result in faulty instructions being given to the cell, the wrong protein being synthesized. Errors of this nature could add up in time to the point of cell division or function being impaired. The accumulation of impairment in different cell types across the body might then translate into what is seen as aging. Altered protein synthesis could also trigger an autoimmune response, with the organism viewing the new protein as a foreign invader. Attacks by the immune system might then weaken the cell, cause it to malfunction, and eventually lead to its death. Reservations about this theory recur with a number of the postulates offered to explain the aging process, namely, that findings have not been demonstrated to be adequate in adding up to the magnitude and variety of recognized age changes.

Caloric Theory/Collagen Theory/Cross-linkage Theory

Heavy caloric intake has been hypothesized to contribute to the aging process (Bjorksten, 1969). It has been suggested that the repeated gorging of 3,300 calories (a common daily intake) in single sittings can lead to the build-up of harmful by-products that interfere with normal cell function. It has also been put forth that heavy diets contribute to abnormal biochemical cross-linkage between cells, impairing the proper activity of the individual cells. By this theory cross-linking could, for example, "clog" glandular cells, thereby impeding critical production and release of hormones and other essential cell products (Hayflick, 1985). Because cross-linkages have been described to occur in the extracellular protein found in the collagenous fibers that normally bind tissues together, this concept has come to be called the collagen theory. Criticisms of this theory point out that there has been no direct evidence to show that cross-linking is either essential or sufficient to explain the changes observed with aging.

The Free Radical Theory

Free radicals are chemical compounds, typically short-lived before changing into a different chemical form, that may be involved as highly active intermediates in various reactions within living tissue (*Stedman's Medical Dictionary,* 1966). The process by which fats become rancid reflects a stepwise progression of free radical reactions. Free radicals consist of an atom or groups of atoms carrying an unpaired electron, the tendency of electrons to pair explaining the nature of the reactivity. Themselves unstable molecules, free radicals can combine sequentially with stable molecules in chain reactions. Such reactions are common as normal physiologic cellular events. Abnormal free radical reactions have been considered to be a source of cell damage in a variety of disease processes (including Alzheimer's disease) and have been theorized to have a role in aging (Hayflick, 1985). Knowledge of the nature of these reactions, however, is not precise. Proponents of this theory postulate that pathological changes occur within both the cell's nucleus and cytoplasm. Inadequate repair processes would then lead to this damage becoming cumulative, resulting in a progressive deterioration in normal functioning. If, for example, DNA in the cell's nucleus became damaged, negative consequences would follow. Faulty proteins could be produced, causing disordered work by the cell. Alternatively, faulty proteins could bring on an autoimmune reaction, as discussed above in the genetic mutation/error theory.

Of further interest with the free radical theory of aging is the purported role of antioxidant compounds in keeping free radical reactions in check. Based on such claims, antioxidants have been used by individuals with the goal of retarding the aging process (their effect will be discussed in more detail below). Doubters of the free radical hypothesis raise the possibility that cell products formed from free radical reactions may be harmless, nondegradable waste substances—lipofuscin perhaps.

The Lipofuscin Theory

Lipofuscin is a pigmented substance found to increase with aging, building up in a diversity of cells, including neurons in the cerebral cortex. While its chemical composition is partially established, its significance is not clear (Hayflick, 1985). Whether it results from intrinsic phenomena, extrinsic factors, or an interplay of the two, is not known. While some speculate that the build-up of this "age pigment" influences aging by interfering with the cell's mitochondria which provide energy and enzymes for critical cell processes, others see it simply as a cellular waste product that has no deleterious effect. In relation to the latter hypothesis it has been referred to as wear-and-tear residue (Brizzee, Ordy, Hofer, & Kaack, 1978). Because lipofuscin has been found in brain cells of those with Alzheimer's disease, it has also been looked at as a potential pathologic influence in this disorder. But, here too, it is not apparent that lipofuscin is anything more than an innocuous waste product, since its accumulation is no greater in Alzheimer patients than in normal age-matched control subjects (Terry, 1985).

Meanwhile, interest in lipofuscin has led to the search for other substances found in cells that may be associated with aging, and thereby offer new clues as to why we age. A newly discovered protein referred to as *statin,* is being studied as possibly representing such a substance (Wang, 1985; Wang & Lin, 1986). Statin is reported to appear late in the life of certain cells, attracting interest in it as a potential biomarker of aging. Its significance, though, remains a research question.

The Immunologic Theory

According to the immunologic theory of normal aging, alterations transpire within the immune system with the passage of time. As a result, immunologic response becomes less efficient, and the organism becomes more vulnerable to infection and general breakdown. A second version of the immunologic theory postulates that cells that cannot divide, for example, cardiac muscle cells and neurons, become increasingly vulnerable to adverse immune system responses over time. Because they exist for a greater period of time, nondividing cells would have more opportunities than dividing ones to develop alterations—changes at increased risk of being misread as foreign bodies and leading to immune system attack (as in the "Error Theory"). According to this second version of the theory, the heart and the brain might be more affected by the aging process, with the frequency of cardiac disorders and the existence of Alzheimer's disease in the elderly attracting attention from an immunologic perspective (Terry & Davies, 1983).

The thymus gland has also been implicated in the aging process in relation to its role in our immune system. Animal studies have shown that removal of the thymus produces deficiencies in immunologic response resembling those seen with aging. To the extent that the thymus gland might influence the time course of immunologic changes, it has been considered as a possible clock of aging (Burnet, 1970).

A major strike against the immune theory of aging comes from its lack of universality; many organisms that age have very rudimentary immune systems, if not lacking them entirely (Hayflick, 1985). Further doubts derive from suggestions that the immune system may be influenced by more fundamental events in the neuroendocrine system, the latter acting as a more basic time keeper.

Clocks of Aging/Theories on Hormones and the Endocrine System

In addition to considerations about the thymus gland acting as a clock of aging and thereby influencing the timing of changes that contribute to the organism becoming physiologically old, other anatomical sites have also been looked at as potential aging clocks or pacemakers of the aging process. The role of the endocrine system in the dramatic physiologic events that accompany growth, maturation, and development throughout the life course has not been overlooked in theories about aging (Finch, 1988). Just as hormones are integrally involved around puberty and menopause, they have been espoused as a catalyst of aging and even death. Terms like "death hormones" have been used in the popular press and other publications on aging from time to time in this regard (Pearson & Shaw, 1982). Historically, there have been many beliefs that use of the right hormone or proper combination of such natural or synthetic substances would delay the course of aging. These attempts have not met with success.

Brain hormone activity, or neuroendocrine physiology, has attracted much interest in efforts to understand the nature of diverse changes throughout the body over time. Attention to the pituitary gland and the hypothalamus in the aging brain have received particular attention as higher control centers of age-related changes. The pituitary gland was initially looked as the pacemaker of the course of growing old, but subsequent research led to the discovery that the hypothalamus played a key role in regulating the pituitary. Hence, the hypothalamus has assumed primacy in pacemaker theories which continue to be under study. The issue of universality, though, has been raised around neuroendocrine considerations, just as it was with the immunologic theory of aging; here, too, not all organisms that age possess neuroendocrine systems with a complexity that would appear necessary to influence the aging process (Hayflick, 1985).

Conclusions from Biological Theories of Aging

Clearly one is not at a loss for theories to explain biologically why we age. For the most part, current theories of aging are not mutually exclusive of one another, and there are problems that challenge the adequacy if not accuracy of each theory (Hayflick, 1985). Researchers have raised the *cause* or *effect* question, wondering whether various phenomena (e.g., immune system changes, neuroendocrine responses, etc.) that have led to separate theories actually reflect a more fundamental process producing the "surface" phenomena. In other words, does the phenomenon described *cause* changes associated with aging, or is this phenomenon itself the *effect* of a more basic factor. At the same time, doubts center on the failure to prove that evidence for various hypotheses is either essential or sufficient to explain the manifestations of aging.

Others, looking at the large number of intriguing (though not proven) theories, have speculated or philosophized that aging is too critical a matter to be left in the hands of one set of determinants—that either an interplay of factors is occurring at molecular, cell, and organ levels to ensure that we will all eventually grow old and die, or that independent processes are operating as de facto backups to make aging and dying inevitable. Interestingly, the search for the cause of Alzheimer's disease has confronted the investigator with a similar complex weave of multiple variables, each implicated in some way with the clinical changes being observed. Meanwhile, the failure to solve the mystery of aging has not interfered with the quest for life extension. Before examining efforts to extend life-span, it would be useful to look at syndromes that shorten longevity—syndromes historically viewed as premature aging and examined with the aim of discovering new clues about the aging process.

PROGERIA

Another approach to discovering why one grows old is to search for conditions where aging seems to have speeded up. There are a few clinical syndromes that have been examined as possible examples of premature aging. They have been lumped together and referred to collectively as *progeria* (from Greek, meaning premature old age) (Brown, 1987; Busse & Blazer, 1980c; Hayflick, 1977; Selmanowitz, Rizer, & Orentreich, 1977). The two types of progeria most commonly discussed are both very rare—the Hutchinson-Gilford syndrome and Werner's syndrome. Although doubts are expressed that these two syndromes represent true examples of accelerated aging, any condition sufficiently resembling aging deserves consideration as a potential source of new insights. Individuals with the Hutchinson-Gilford syndrome can display by age 10 physical signs associated with aging among persons over 70. These progerics look old and wizened, with loss of hair, eyebrows, and eyelashes. Their disorder is characterized by dwarfism and generalized atherosclerosis affecting all major blood vessels. They generally die of coronary artery disease before reaching 20 years of age. The syndrome occurs in both sexes and several races and is believed to be an inherited state caused by an autosomal recessive trait.

Werner's syndrome has a later onset (between the ages of 15 and 20) than the Hutchinson-Gilford syndrome, but otherwise physically resembles it with the prematurely old and wizened appearance of affected individuals. Those with Werner's syndrome have an average life expectancy of 47 years, and manifest short stature, thin limbs, a beak-shaped nose, receding chin, juvenile cataracts, proneness to diabetes, osteoporosis, atherosclerosis, and calcification of blood vessels, and a high incidence of malignancy. Relevant to the discussion of cell death as a theory of aging above, those with Werner's syndrome have shown a striking decrease in the normal number of cell doublings; this is apparently not the case with the Hutchinson-Gilford syndrome. Like the Hutchinson-Gilford syndrome, Werner's syndrome is also believed to be an hereditary condition transmitted by an autosomal recessive trait. There has been a report of consanguineous marriages being associated with a large number of those who developed Werner's syndrome in one sample studied.

To date the different forms of progeria have not contributed important information leading to a better understanding of the aging process. While certain features of these syndromes seem akin to those associated with normal aging, other normal concomitants of the aging process are entirely lacking. For example, in the Hutchinson-Gilford syndrome, findings inconsistent with aging include delayed dentition, no increase in the incidence of tumors, and no elevation in tissue lipofuscin levels; in Werner's syndrome, sexual maturity is delayed (Tice & Setlow, 1985). Brain studies of those with progeria are largely lacking. Senile dementia has not been reported. With the Hutchinson-Gilford syndrome it has been reported that a few individuals have been mentally retarded, though most have been described as having normal intelligence or even being precocious (*Encyclopaedia Britannica,* 1985a).

LIFE EXTENSION AND REJUVENATION

From primitive societies to the present there has been a continued quest for prescriptions for rejuvenation and life extension (Bailey, 1987; de Beauvoir, 1978; Freeman, 1979). Emphasis is placed on prolonging one's years and in restoring vitality to the aging brain, body, and libido. The earliest written formulas are found in the *Ebers papyrus,* an Egyptian compilation of medical information dating back to around 1550–1800 B.C., representing one of the oldest known medical works. This famous scroll was noted for the number of remedies it offered—more than 700, ranging from the treatment of crocodile bite to ridding the house of scorpions. Out of the golden age of Indian medicine dating from around 800 B.C. until about 1000 A.D. emerged ideas expressed in the work of Sushruta, which was finally published around the 7th century A.D. Sushruta's prescriptions included soma, a mountain plant that was likely valued for its exhilarating, probably hallucinogenic effect. In the 15th century, Pope Innocent VIII sought rejuvenation through receiving a transfusion of the blood of young men into his veins; he died almost immediately, most likely from incompatible blood types.

The Renaissance movement witnessed the image of restorative waters becoming more vivid, reviving the 700 B.C. Hindu hope to find the *Pool of Youth* (Gruman, 1966). Cranach the Elder painted the *Fons Juventutis,* the fountain of youth, and his contemporary Juan Ponce de Leon began his legendary 16th century search for the same. While Ponce de Leon did not locate the mythical fountain, he did discover Florida, the warm waters of which have attracted retirement living for many aging individuals. In the 18th century all of Europe knew of the prescription of the famed Dutch physician and professor of medicine, Hermann Boerhaave, for an old man to sleep between two virginal young women to regain health (the anticipated outcome for the two women was not made clear). Boerhaave's approach actually dated back to biblical times and an intervention described for King David in the Bible in the First Book of Kings (1 Kings, 1:2): "Let them seek out for my lord the king a young virgin, and let her stand before the king, and let her be an attendant on him; and let her lie in thy bosom, that my lord the king may become warm." The early Greeks and Romans also adopted this approach and described the restorative factor as the "quality of a virgin's breath," the technique itself coming to be called "gerokomy" (Guillerme, 1963). By the end of the 19th century, proximity to virgins' breaths had given way to injections of testicular extracts as the leading prescription for increased longevity (McGrady, 1968). In 1889 no less a figure than the noted French physiologist and Harvard professor Brown-Séquard injected himself with extract from sheep testicles, claiming it took 30 years off his age. Though six feet four inches in height, Brown-Séquard subsequently suffered somewhat in scientific stature.

During the early part of the 20th century, the Russian born surgeon Serge Voronoff moved from injecting extracts from testicles to grafting testicles themselves in attempts to restore youth to aging men. Voronoff is reported to have carried out over 2,000 such operations. However, he neglected advice from colleagues who recommended that his donors be bulls. Instead, Voronoff grafted monkey testicles, asserting that since man is a primate, the procedure would be more successful by using other primates (e.g., monkeys or apes) as donors. Monkeys, however, are much more likely than bulls to transmit venereal disease to man. As a result, in addition to numerous problems with immunologic rejection of the grafts, many of the subjects also contracted syphilis (McGrady, 1968).

As the 20th century advanced, mixed heritages from alchemy and medicine in an historical backdrop of elixors, potions, and tonics converged in the search for the restorative pill. Gerovital-H_3, a procaine hydrochloride derivative, was seen as such a candidate. Procaine hydrochloride had been used in various tonics in Europe since the early 1900s. Then in the 1940s, Professor Anna Aslan of the Geriatric Institute of Bucharest, Romania began to report a variety of positive effects on problems associated with aging, from improved skin texture to better memory. Since then Gerovital has crossed the Atlantic, where a series of studies, replicated in Britain, found the drug not to be effective in altering negative changes associated with aging (Davison, 1978).

With the above as background, a more detailed review of major recent approaches to extending life and retarding the aging process will be reviewed. *In no case* is there evidence that any of these approaches influences the aging process per se in humans (Masoro, 1987; Schneider & Reed,

1985). An intervention can influence life expectancy without affecting life-span (Hayflick, 1985; Masoro, 1987; Schneider & Reed, 1985). The difference between these two terms is more than semantic and highly relevant to this discussion. Life expectancy indicates the average number of years a member of a given species would normally live (e.g., approximately 75 years for Americans in 1985). Life-span designates the maximum age a member of that species might possibly reach (thought to be approximately 115 years in humans). Life-span is more fundamentally linked to the process of aging itself, while life expectancy is significantly influenced by factors beyond aging alone; such as disease, war, and famine. This is why average life expectancy has varied so enormously over the centuries, but not life-span.

To demonstrate unequivocally that an intervention alters the process of aging, one would have to show that life-span can be increased; to date this has not been accomplished in humans. Life expectancy, on the other hand, is continuously being altered by advances in medicine. Antibiotics that treat pneumonia in an older person increase that individual's life expectancy, but not his or her life-span. One group of critics contends that if an approach to life extension has an effect, its influence is on life expectancy, probably by altering some underlying process that influences illness. Nonetheless, this would be no small accomplishment in terms of prevention of age-related diseases. Another group of critics doubts that many of the approaches prescribed have any effect at all. Finally, most of the positive results reported in this area of research come from studies on laboratory animals, with relatively little rigorous data on people. Still, investigators in this area remain largely undaunted. A number of the major current approaches follows.

Exercise and Longevity

In laboratory animals, exercise begun early in life and continued throughout the life course has been found to increase both life expectancy and life-span. Exercise started in later life has not had a clear effect on extending survival in these animals. In humans it is difficult to identify studies of lifelong exercise. There have been studies, though, that have looked at the longevity of those who were athletes in college. One such study compared the life expectancies of nearly 5,000 former collegiate athletes with nearly 40,000 graduates in general from the same universities. No difference was found between the life expectancies of the two groups (Shock, 1977). Another study compared the longevity of lettermen (more accomplished athletes) with three different groups of nonathletes who had attended college. In none of these comparisons did the athletic group outlive the others. Moreover, those in the control groups who had achieved scholastic honors had on the average a two-year greater longevity than both the athletes and the general group of nonathletes (Polednak & Damon, 1970). Perhaps this speaks to how individuals use their brains as well as their bodies as they age. Though there is no evidence that those who are athletically active early on in life live any longer than those who are not, we do not have enough information to reach conclusions about the effect of more prolonged formal exercise.

On the other hand, a number of studies have demonstrated the beneficial effects of exercise on various disorders that increase in frequency as we age, ranging from retarding bone mineral loss that can contribute to osteoporosis to slowing decremental changes in cardiovascular performance (and lowering the risk for coronary artery disease) (Paffenbarger, Hyde, Wing, & Steinmetz, 1984; Schneider, 1985). The latter may have relevance to preserving intellectual performance with advancing age given the greater likelihood of decrements in cognitive functioning in those who develop cardiovascular disease as opposed to those who do not (Granick & Patterson, 1972).

Restriction of Calories and Longevity

Attention to the relationship of diet to longevity and to the quality of aging is not new. In 1534, for example, the famous for its time *Castel of Helthe,* a popular regimen of health, contained important dietary advice for the elderly; it was written by Sir Thomas Elyot, a member of Sir Thomas More's circle and noted for his breadth of knowledge in literature, philosophy, and medicine. Elyot's admonitions to the aging included that of a prudent diet: "Always remember that aged men should eat often; and but little every time, for it fareth by them as it doth by a lamp, the light whereof is almost extinct, which by pouring oil and little is kept long burning, but with much oil poured in at once, it is put out" (Freeman, 1979, p. 36).

Since the 1930s it has been recognized that restricting calories while supplementing essential nutrients to laboratory rats extends both their life expectancy and their life-span (Sacher, 1977). Why this should occur is not understood. Other than some reports that restricting calories curtails collagen cross-linking—connecting it to a theory of aging alluded to above—explanations remain sketchy. It does appear that caloric restriction reduces the frequency or delays the onset in these animals of various diseases, including tumors, respiratory disease, and renal disorders. Thus, caloric levels may reduce morbidity caused by age-related illnesses, thereby prolonging life in a secondary manner. But here, too, a mechanism of action is elusive. It has also been pointed out that the severe caloric restriction required for maximal life extension in rodents *retards growth* and consequently becomes an undesirable intervention for humans

(Schneider & Reed, 1985). Moreover, it has been suggested that rats in their natural habitat eat on an irregular schedule, the outcome of which could correspond to laboratory conditions of caloric restriction. In other words, restricting calories in the safe environment of the lab might be akin to a more typical eating pattern of rodents in their natural environment confronting everyday threats that disrupt diets.

The significance of restricting calories has not been that of controlling obesity in these longevity studies. Typically animals of normal weight have been examined in this research. Obesity, of course, is an issue in its own right as a risk factor in aggravating various disorders. On the other hand, one has to watch out that weight control does not result in undernutrition, that is, not getting enough of the essential vitamins and minerals due to an inadequate, unbalanced diet. The elderly and the aging brain require more careful attention to these needs. Certain nutritional deficiencies can have serious consequences for cerebral functioning in old age (Exton-Smith & Overstall, 1979). Vitamin B deficiencies have long been known to cause such problems. For the most part when vitamin deficiencies do occur with the elderly, they are precipitated not by normal aging, but by an associated disease state. Thiamine (vitamin B_1) deficiency, for example, which can cause Korsakoff's dementia, is associated with chronic alcohol abuse and accompanying poor nutritional behavior. In the absence of an underlying pathologic process in the elderly, vitamin deficiencies appear not to be a problem (Barrows & Roeder, 1977).

The Effect of Vitamin E and Dietary Antioxidants on Free Radicals and Longevity

Based on the free radical theory of aging described above, antioxidants have been used in efforts to halt or slow free radical chain reactions and thereby alter the process of aging. Studies with laboratory animals do show that antioxidants can prolong their lives (Kohn, 1971; Sanadi, 1977). It has also been noted, though, that in a number of these studies unanticipated weight loss occurred in conjunction, making the results more difficult to interpret in the context of caloric reduction as just discussed (Schneider & Reed, 1985). One should be reminded, too, of the caution about generalizing findings from animal research to conclusions about human populations.

Because Vitamin E is a very potent natural antioxidant, it has attracted particular attention in studies on both the aging brain and the aging body as a whole (Blackett & Hall, 1981; Brody & Vijayashankar, 1977). Interestingly, the deposition of lipofuscin appears to increase in conjunction with vitamin E deficiency, but supplementing vitamin E has not been found to either inhibit lipofuscin accumulation or to extend longevity (Hayflick,

1985). Vitamins C and A as well as the mineral selenium have also been promoted by some and doubted by others to be of value in life extension (Ames, 1983; Willet & MacMahon, 1984). An important review of these substances reported the following conclusions (Schneider & Reed, 1985):

> Although the possible antineoplastic and anti-aging actions of vitamins A, C, and E and of the mineral selenium deserve further investigation, the available evidence at this time does not support recommending diet supplementation with these vitamins or selenium for either life extension or the prevention of cancer. It is of interest that studies of vitamin consumption by a highly selected group of people (pooled readers of *Prevention* magazine) over age 65 found no dose–response relationship between mortality and the levels of vitamin supplementation. In this same study, increased mortality was observed in people who consumed very high levels of vitamin E—more than 1000 IU per day. Although this last observation may reflect the attraction for less healthy persons of large doses of vitamins, it may also reflect some vitamin toxicity. Thus, caution is advised before the ingestion of large doses of these vitamins or selenium is considered. (p. 1161)

The Effect of Centrophenoxine on the Age Pigment Lipofuscin and Longevity

There have been attempts to test the lipofuscin theory of aging by applying chemicals, apart from vitamin E, for the purpose of decreasing the amount of the age pigment deposited in the body's tissues. If lipofuscin does cause aging, then drugs that lower the level of the pigment should alter some of the changes seen with aging, prolong life, or both. Centrophenoxine® (also known as meclofenoxate, Clofenoxine®, Helfergin®, Lucidril®, and ANP 235) has been the most widely used drug for this purpose. In a variety of laboratory animals centrophenoxine has been reported to decrease the accumulation of lipofuscin (Nandy & Bourne, 1966; Riga & Riga, 1974), and in other such studies to prolong life (Schneider & Reed, 1985). There have also been studies of centrophenoxine in humans, where its usage was followed by reduced fasting blood sugar levels, increased maximal oxygen consumption, and weight loss—the latter raising again the potential role of caloric reduction in explaining observed changes (Schneider & Reed, 1985). Global changes relevant to the aging process, however, have not been reported in people.

Less globally, centrophenoxine's effect on the aging brain of Alzheimer patients is being examined. One of the consistent findings in Alzheimer's disease research has been reduced brain levels of the neurotransmitter acetylcholine. Centrophenoxine has been looked at as a potential precursor of choline which is involved in the synthesis of acetylcholine. By administering centrophenoxine to those with Alzheimer's disease investigators have hoped to elevate acetylcholine levels and thereby improve memory functioning. To date, results have not been clinically significant (Bartus, Dean, Flicker, & Beer, 1983; Goodnick & Gershon, 1983).

Immunologic Approaches to Longevity

With a finger pointed at the immune system as playing a possible part in the aging process, manipulations of the immune system have been attempted to study the impact on aging. These efforts have been referred to as "immunoengineering" (Makinodan, 1977). Dietary restriction is one approach that has been tried in animals, with the result of reducing certain autoimmune phenomena in laboratory mice (Fernande, Yunis, Jose, & Good, 1973). Life-span was increased in some studies on laboratory animals, though this may have been due to strengthening the immune system against disease, as opposed to a direct effect on the aging process.

Deterioration in the functioning of the thymus having been implicated in various age-related changes has led to attempts to transplant compatible thymic cells from young animal donors to old recipients. While these grafts have decreased the formation of autoantibodies seen in mice with aging and have improved specific immune functions in the aged mice, no effect on life-span was witnessed (Schneider & Reed, 1985). Similar results occurred with the grafting of other immune cells in laboratory animals.

Pharmacologic agents have also been used in attempts to rejuvenate the immune system and the organism as a whole. Referred to as adjuvants— chemicals which nonspecifically promote normal immune activities— these drugs have varied from vitamin E as mentioned above to a group of coenzymes known collectively as coenzymes Q (Makinodan, 1977; Schneider & Reed, 1985). Coenzyme Q_{10} has been reported on the one hand to protect mice from viral and carcinogen-induced tumor formation, but on the other hand to have damaging effects on various tissues. The need to explore for toxic responses while seeking beneficial effects continues to come up in the various studies of substances ingested in the hope of promoting improved aging or life extension.

Hormone Manipulation and Longevity

During the 1920s and 1930s popular as well as medical publications contained numerous accounts of the rejuvenating power of "gland" therapy, as hormones were administered in the hope of restoring youth. Virtually none of that work has been validated (Sacher, 1977). Moreover, many of these hormone treatments were not without negative consequences in the form of various growths that were stimulated in aging tissues. In addition to adding hormones, the earlier alluded to concept of "death hormones" led to efforts to remove organs suspected of harboring the offenders. The pituitary in particular came under the knife in laboratory animals. Aging rats that had their pituitary removed were reported to have had reduced collagen cross-linking, delayed thymic involution, and fewer age-related changes in their vasculature, kidneys, and immune system. In addition, a familiar confounding change occurred—weight loss pointing to food restriction, with the potential role of reduced caloric intake influencing all these changes (Schneider & Reed, 1985). Regardless, removal of the pituitary is not without negative consequences, such as in stunting skeletal growth (Tonna, 1977).

Conclusions from Efforts at Life Extension

As attempting to find the cause of aging has not been easy, it should not be surprising that a sure formula for life extension has been similarly elusive. Furthermore, just as some have suggested that aging may well be the outcome of a combination of events, others have likewise speculated that any possibility of life extension would probably depend on more than a single isolated approach. In the interim, some of the results from the research on prolonging life could lead to more effective approaches to reducing some of the age-related illnesses, thereby improving the quality if not the duration of later life.

From a different perspective, while difficulty in identifying what causes us to age may leave us frustrated, efforts to achieve life extension may be met with more serious consequences—such as risks of negative effects if drugs or experimental techniques are involved. The metaphor of the good news/bad news situation might be good to keep in mind. Meanwhile, in the search for answers about aging and leads to life extension, hopefully the ancient myth of Tithonous (whom the gods gave immortality without controlling for aging) will not be repeated and we will be able to reduce frailty while struggling with the concept of finality.

Appendixes

Appendix A.1

Suggested Criteria for Clinical Diagnosis of Alzheimer's Disease*

I. The criteria for the clinical diagnosis of probable Alzheimer's disease include:

- dementia established by clinical examination and documented by the Mini-Mental Scale, Blessed Dementia Scale, or some similar examination, and possibly confirmed by neuropsychological tests
- deficits in two or more areas of cognition; progressive worsening of memory and other cognitive functions
- no disturbance of consciousness
- onset between ages 40 and 90, most often after age 65
- absence of systemic disorders or other brain diseases that in and of themselves could account for the progressive deficits in memory cognition.

II. The diagnosis of probable Alzheimer's disease is supported by:

- progressive deterioration of specific cognitive functions such as language (aphasia), motor skills (apraxia), and perception (agnosia)
- impaired activities of daily living and altered patterns of behavior
- family history of similar disorders, particularly if confirmed neuropathologically

* This Appendix was adapted from McKhann et al. (1984).

- laboratory results of:
    normal lumbar puncture as evaluated by standard techniques
    normal pattern or nonspecific changes in EEG, such as increased
        slow wave activity
    evidence of cerebral atrophy on CT with progression documented
        by serial observation.

III. Other clinical features consistent with the diagnosis of probable Alzheimer's disease, after exclusion of causes of dementia other than Alzheimer's disease, include:

- plateaus in the course of progression of the illness
- associated symptoms such as depression, insomnia, incontinence, delusions, illusions, hallucinations, catastrophic verbal, emotional, or physical outbursts, sexual disorders, and weight loss
- other neurological abnormalities in some patients, especially with more advanced disease and including motor signs such as increased muscle tone, myoclonus, or gait disorder
- seizures in advanced disease
- CT normal for age.

IV. Features that make the diagnosis of probable Alzheimer's disease uncertain or unlikely include:

- sudden apoplectic onset
- focal neurologic findings such as hemiparesis, sensory loss, visual field deficits, and incoordination early in the course of the illness
- seizures or gait disturbances at the onset or very early in the course of the illness.

V. Clinical diagnosis of possible Alzheimer's disease:

- may be made on the basis of the dementia syndrome in the absence of other neurologic, psychiatric, or systemic disorders sufficient to cause dementia, and in the presence of variations in the onset, in the presentation, or in the clinical course
- may be made in the presence of a second systemic or brain disorder sufficient to produce dementia which is not considered to be the cause of the dementia
- should be used in research studies when a single, gradually progressive severe cognitive deficit is identified in the absence of other identifiable cause.

VI. Criteria for diagnosis of definite Alzheimer's disease are:

- the clinical criteria for probable Alzheimer's disease
- histopathologic evidence obtained from a biopsy or autopsy.

VII. Classification of Alzheimer's disease for research purposes should specify features that may differentiate subtypes of the disorder, such as:

- familial occurrence
- onset before age of 65
- presence of trisomy-21
- coexistence of other relevant conditions such as Parkinson's disease.

Appendix A.2

Tests for the Differential Diagnosis of Dementing Disorders*

The best diagnostic test is a careful history and physical and mental status examination.

The laboratory tests that are used should be individualized based on the history and physical and mental status examination. Overtesting may expose the patient to discomfort, inconvenience, excess costs, and the likelihood of false positive tests that may lead to additional unnecessary testing. Undertesting also has hazards, for example, in elderly persons, where medical disease may have nonspecific presentations such as dementia.

All patients with new onset of dementia should have several basic and standard diagnostic studies, with modifications to be made according to individual circumstances:

1. Complete blood count.
2. Electrolyte panel.
3. Screening metabolic panel.

* This Appendix is adapted from the National Institutes of Health Consensus Development Conference Statement on the Differential Diagnosis of Dementing Diseases, 1987.

4. Thyroid function studies.
5. Vitamin B_{12} and folate levels.
6. Tests for syphilis and, depending on history, for human immunodeficiency antibodies.
7. Urinalysis.
8. Electrocardiogram.
9. Chest x-ray.

Most of the readily reversible metabolic, endocrine, deficiency, and infectious states, whether causative or complicating, will be revealed by these simple investigations when combined with history and physical examination.

Other ancillary studies are appropriate in certain common situations:

1. Computed tomography of the brain (without contrast) is appropriate in the presence of history suggestive of a mass, or focal neurologic signs, or in dementia of brief duration. Unless such diagnosis is obvious on first contact, computed tomography should be done.

2. All medications that are not absolutely necessary should be discontinued.

3. Electroencephalograms are appropriate for patients with altered consciousness or suspected seizure, depending on the clinical circumstances.

4. Formal psychiatric assessment is desirable when depression is suspected.

5. Inpatient hospitalization should be considered when the history is unclear, if the patient is suicidal, when an acute deterioration has occurred without apparent cause, or if the social situation precludes adequate observation.

6. Neuropsychological evaluation is appropriate (1) to obtain baseline information against which to measure change in cases in which diagnosis is in doubt, (2) before and following treatment, (3) in cases of exceptionally bright individuals suspected of early dementia, (4) in cases of ambiguous imaging findings that require elucidation, (5) to help distinguish dementia from depression and delirium, and (6) to provide additional information about the extent and nature of impairment following focal or multifocal brain injury.

7. Speech and language analysis can be very helpful. In some patients, complex language disorders can simulate dementia; in others, the skillful speech pathologist can help the patient and family to communicate better.

The role of other studies is controversial, and firm rules for their routine use are not appropriate. Undue weight should not be placed on isolated laboratory findings unless they are consistent with previous clinical information. Examples of these other studies include the following:

1. Magnetic resonance imaging is more sensitive than computed tomography for detection of small infarcts, mass lesions, atrophy of the brainstem, and other subcortical structures; it also may clarify ambiguous computed tomography findings. Inexperienced interpreters may make too much of ambiguous or nonspecific findings on magnetic resonance imaging.

2. Regional cerebral blood flow and metabolism measurements (positron emission tomography and single photon emission computed tomography) are research techniques that have no proven *routine* clinical value at the present time. Their value in predicting Huntington's and Alzheimer's disease in individuals at risk is under investigation.

3. Lumbar puncture is not routinely required in the initial evaluation of dementia. It should be performed when other clinical findings suggest an active infection or vasculitis. At present, cerebrospinal fluid markers for Alzheimer's disease are not sufficiently well developed to justify routine lumbar puncture.

4. Electrophysiological techniques such as event-related potentials that are recorded using special electroencephalographic techniques are not recommended for routine use.

5. Brain biopsy for nontumorous and noninfectious diseases rarely is justified except in a small number of unusual clinical situations.

6. Biological markers for progressive degenerative dementing disease are still in the investigative stage. Although some give promise, they are not ready for widespread or routine use.

7. Significant major findings have been made on the molecular genetics of conditions like Huntington's and Alzheimer's diseases, but these findings have restricted usefulness at present.

8. Carotid ultrasound is of no value except sometimes in the search for the cause of infarcts.

Appendix **A.3**

Antidepressant Drugs*

Generic name	Usual geriatric dose range (mg/day)	Sedation potential	Potential for hypotension	Potential for cardiac side effects	Anti-cholinergic potential
Tricyclic antidepressants					
Amitriptyline	50–100	+++	++	+++	+++/++++
Trimipramine	50–100	+++	++	+++	+++
Imipramine	30–100	+	++	++	++/+++
Doxepin	25–100	++/+++	++	++	+++/++++
Protriptyline	15–20	+	++	++	+++
Nortriptyline	30–50	+	+	+	++
Desipramine	25–100	+	+/++	+	+
New generation antidepressants					
Amoxapine	75–150	+	++	++	++
Maprotiline	50–75	++/+++	++	+	++
Trazadone	50–150	+++/++++	++	+/++	−/+

Key: − indicates absent; + indicates mild; ++ indicates moderate; +++ indicates severe; ++++ indicates very severe; / indicates in between (hence, −/+ indicates absent to mild).

Adapted from: DiGiacomo and Prien (1983), Nickens, Crook, and Cohen (1986), and Salzman (1984c).

Appendix A.4

Antipsychotic Drugs: Dosage and Side Effect Comparisons*

Generic name	Usual geriatric dose range (mg/day)	Equivalent dosage in mg/100 mg chlorpromazine	Sedation potential	Potential for hypotension	Potential for anti-cholinergic side effects	Potential for extra-pyramidal side effects
Chlorpromazine	10–300	100	+++	+++	+++	++
Chlorprothixene	10–300	100	+++	+++	+++	++
Thioridazine	10–300	100	+++	+++	++	+/++
Acetophenazine	10–60	19	++	++	++	++
Perphenazine	4–32	10	++	++	++	++
Loxapine	5–100	10	++	++	++	++
Molindone	5–100	10	++	++	++	++
Thiothixene	4–20	5	++	++	++/+	++/+++
Trifluperazine	4–20	5	++	++	++/+	++/+++
Fluphenazine	0.25–6	2	+	+	+	+++
Haloperidol	0.25–6	2	+	+	+	+++

Key: + indicates mild; ++ indicates moderate; +++ indicates marked; / indicates in between (hence, +/++ indicates mild to moderate).

Equivalent dosage: Comparing haloperidol to chlorpromazine on the table, one finds that 2 mg haloperidol is the equivalent in potency to 100 mg chlorpromazine.

*Adapted from: Davis (1981) and Salzman (1984c).

Appendix A.5

Antianxiety Drugs: Dosages and Half-Life Characteristics*

Generic name	Usual geriatric dose range (mg/day)	Young adults (hr)	Older adults (hr)
	Long acting		
Diazepam	2–20	24	75
Chlordiazepoxide	5–40	10	30
	Intermediate acting		
Alprazolam	0.25–2	10	17
	Short acting		
Lorazepam	0.5–4	12	12
Oxazepam	10–40	10	10

Note: A half-life is the amount of time that it takes half the amount of the drug ingested to be deactivated or removed from the body.

Adapted from: Salzman (1982) and Salzman (1984c).

References

Abraham, K. (1979). Applicability of psycho-analytic treatment to patients at an advanced age. In H. C. Abraham (Ed.), *Selected papers on psychoanalysis.* New York: Brunner/Mazel.

Adams, R. D. (1980). The morphological aspects of aging in the human nervous system. In J. E. Birren, & R. B. Sloane (Eds.), *Handbook of mental health and aging.* Englewood Cliffs, NJ: Prentice-Hall.

Age Page. (1988). Report outlines findings and potential breakthroughs in aging research. *Neurobiology of Aging, 9,* 145.

Alexander, F. G., & Selesnic, S. T. (1966). *The history of psychiatry.* New York: Harper & Row.

Alpaugh, P. K., Parham, I. A., Cole, K. D., & Birren, J. E. (1982). Creativity in adulthood and old age: An exploratory study. *Educational Gerontology 8:* 101–116.

Alzheimer, A. (1907). Uber eine eigenartige erkrankung der hirnrinde. *Allg. Z. Psychiatrie Psychisch-Gerichtlich. Med., 64,* 146–148.

American Psychiatric Association. (1987). *Diagnostic and statistical manual of mental disorders* (3rd ed., rev.). Washington, DC: American Psychiatric Association.

Ames, B. N. (1983). Dietary carcinogens and anticarcinogens: Oxygen radicals and degenerative diseases. *Science, 221,* 1256–1264.

Anderson, J. R. C. (1968). An epilogue. In F. C. Chichester, *Gypsy moth circles the world.* New York: Coward-McCann.

Andreasen, N. C. (1988). Brain imaging: Applications in psychiatry. *Science, 239,* 1381–1388.

Asimov, I. (1965). *The human brain.* New York: A Mentor Book.

Azmitia, E. C., & Bjorklund, A. (1987). Cell and tissue transplantation into the adult brain. *Neurobiology of Aging, 8,* 77–82.

Babigian, H. M. (1985). Schizophrenia: Epidemiology. In H. I. Kaplan, & B. J. Sadock (Eds.), *Comprehensive textbook of psychiatry/IV* (Vol. 1). Baltimore, MD: Williams & Wilkins.

Backlund, E., Granberg, P., Hamberger, B., Knutsson, E., Mårtensson, A., Sedvall, G., Seiger, Å., & Olson, L. (1985). Transplantation of adrenal medullary tissue to striatum in parkinsonism. *Journal of Neurosurgery, 62,* 169–173.

Bailey, E. B. (1967). *James Hutton: The founder of modern geology.* New York: Elsevier Science.

Bailey, W. G. (1987). *Human longevity from antiquity to the modern lab: A selected, annotated bibliography.* New York: Greenwood Press.

Barnes, D. M. (1987). Alzheimer protein is also in infant brains. *Science, 238,* 1652.

Barrett, T. R., & Watkins, S. K. (1986). Word familiarity and cardiovascular health as determinants of age-related recall differences. *Journal of Gerontology, 41* (2), 222–224.

Barrows, C. H., & Roeder, L. M., (1977). Nutrition. In C. E. Finch, & L. Hayflick (Eds.), *Handbook of the biology of aging* (1st ed.). New York: Van Nostrand Reinhold.

Bartus, R. T., Dean, R. L., Flicker, C., & Beer, B. (1983). Behavioral and pharmacological studies using animal models of aging: Implications for studying and treating dementia of Alzheimer's type. In R. Katzman (Ed.), *Biological aspects of Alzheimer's disease* (Banbury Report 15). Cold Spring Harbor, NY: Cold Spring Harbor Laboratory.

Beck, E. M. (Ed.). (1980). *Barlett's familiar quotations.* Boston: Little, Brown and Company.

Bennett, N. G., & Garson, L. K. (1986). Extraordinary longevity in the Soviet Union: Fact or artifact. *The Gerontologist, 26* (4), 359–366.

Berezin, M. A. (1963). Some intrapsychic aspects of aging. In N. E. Zinberg, & I. Kaufman (Eds.), *Normal psychology of the aging process.* New York: International Universities Press.

Berezin, M. A. (1972). Psychodynamic considerations of the aging and the aged: An overview. *American Journal of Psychiatry, 128,* 1483–1491.

Bergmann, K. (1978). Neurosis and personality disorder in old age. In A. D. Isaacs, & F. Post (Eds.), *Studies in geriatric psychiatry.* New York: John Wiley.

Bergmann, K., & Eastman, E. J. (1974). Psychogeriatric ascertainment and assessment for treatment in an acute medical ward setting. *Age and Ageing, 3,* 174–188.

Berkowitz, H., Reichel, J., & Shim, C. (1973). The effect of ethanol on the cough reflex. *Clinical Science and Molecular Medicine, 45,* 527–531.

Berwick, R. (1983). *How to train your pet like a television star.* Los Angeles: Armstrong Publishing Co.

Besedovsky, H. O., DelRey, A. E., & Sorkin, E. (1985). Immune-neuroendocrine interactions. *The Journal of Immunology, 135,* 750s–754s.

Bierman, E. L. (1985). Arteriosclerosis and aging. In C. E. Finch, & E. L. Schneider (Eds.), *Handbook of the biology of aging* (2nd ed.). New York: Van Nostrand Reinhold.

Binstock, R. H. (1985). Health care of the aging: trends, dilemmas, and prospects for the year 2000. In C. M. Gaitz, & T. Samorajski (Eds.), *Aging 2000: our health care destiny, volume I: biomedical issues.* New York: Springer-Verlag.

Birren, J. E., & Bengtson, V. L. (Eds.). (1988). *Emergent theories of aging.* New York: Springer Publishing Co.

Birren, J. E., Butler, R. N., Greenhouse, S. W., Sokoloff, L., & Yarrow, M. R. (Eds.). (1974). *Human aging I: A biological and behavioral study* (DHEW

Publication No. (ADM) 74–122). Rockville, MD: National Institute of Mental Health.

Birren, J. E., & Renner, V. J. (1980). Concepts and issues of mental health and aging. In J. E. Birren, & R. B. Sloane (Eds.), *Handbook of mental health and aging*. Englewood Cliffs, NJ: Prentice-Hall.

Birren, J. E., & Sloane, R. B. (Eds.). (1980). *Handbook of mental health and aging*. Englewood Cliffs, NJ: Prentice-Hall.

Bjorksten, J. (1969). Theories. In S. Bakerman (Ed.), *Aging life processes*. Springfield, IL: Charles C. Thomas.

Blackett, A. D., & Hall, D. A. (1981). Vitamin E—Its significance in mouse ageing. *Age and Ageing, 10,* 191–195.

Blazer, D. (1986). Depression. *Generations, 10,* 21–23.

Blazer, D. G., Bachar, J. R., & Manton, K. G. (1986). Suicide in late life: Review and commentary. *Journal of the American Geriatrics Society, 34,* 519–525.

Blazer, D., Hughes, D. C., & George, L. K. (1987). The epidemiology of depression in an elderly community population. *The Gerontologist, 27* (3), 281–287.

Bleuler, M. (1974). The long-term course of the schizophrenic psychoses. *Psychological Medicine, 4,* 244–254.

Blum, J. E., & Tross, S. (1980). Psychodynamic treatment of the elderly: A review of issues in theory and practice. In C. Eisdorfer (Ed.), *Annual review of gerontology and geriatrics*. New York: Springer Publishing Co.

Boorson, S., Barnes, R. A., Kukull, W. A., et al. (1986). Symptomatic depression in elderly medical outpatients. *Journal of the American Geriatrics Society, 34,* 341–347.

Bridge, T. P., Cannon, H. E., & Wyatt, R. J. (1978). Burned-out schizophrenia: Evidence for age effects on schizophrenic symptomatology. *Journal of Gerontology, 33,* 835–839.

Bridge, T. P., & Wyatt, R. J. (1980a). Paraphrenia: Paranoid states of late life. I: European research. *Journal of the American Geriatrics Society, 28,* 193–200.

Bridge, T. P., & Wyatt, R. J. (1980b). Paraphrenia: Paranoid states of late life. II: American research. *Journal of the American Geriatrics Society, 28,* 201–205.

Briley, M., Chopin, P., & Moret, C. (1986). New concepts in Alzheimer's disease. *Neurobiology of Aging, 7* (1), 57–62.

Brizzee, K. R., Ordy, J. M., Hofer, H., & Kaack, B. (1978). Animal models for the study of senile brain disease and aging changes in the brain. In R. Katzman, R. D. Terry, & K. L. Bick (Eds.), *Alzheimer's disease: Senile dementia and related disorders (Aging,* Vol. 7). New York: Raven Press.

Britannica. (1985a). Aging and senescence. *The New Encyclopaedia Britannica* (Vol. 20). Chicago: Encyclopaedia Britannica.

Britannica. (1985b). Creativity. *The New Encyclopaedia Britannica* (Vol. 3). Chicago: Encyclopaedia Britannica.

Britannica. (1985c). France, Anatole. *The New Encyclopaedia Britannica* (Vol. 4). Chicago: Encyclopaedia Britannica.

Britannica. (1985d). Progeria. *The New Encyclopaedia Britannica* (Vol. 9). Chicago: Encyclopaedia Britannica.

Britannica (1985e). Sanders, Harland. *The New Encyclopaedia Britannica* (Vol. 10). Chicago: Encyclopaedia Britannica.

Britannica. (1985f). Uniformitarianism. *The New Encyclopaedia Britannica* (Vol. 12). Chicago: Encyclopaedia Britannica.

Brody, E. M. (1981). The formal support network: congregate treatment settings for residents with senescent brain dysfunction. In N. E. Miller, & G. D. Cohen

(Eds.), *Clinical aspects of Alzheimer's disease and senile dementia.* New York: Raven Press.

Brody, E. M. (1986). Informal supports systems in the rehabilitation of the disabled elderly. In S. J. Brody, & G. E. Ruff (Eds.), *Aging and rehabilitation.* New York: Springer Publishing Co.

Brody, H. (1978). Cell counts in cerebral cortex and brainstem. In R. Katzman, R. D. Terry, & K. L. Bick (Eds.), *Alzheimer's disease: Senile dementia and related disorders (Aging,* Vol. 7). New York: Raven Press.

Brody, H. (1987). Central nervous system. In G. L. Maddox (Ed.), *The encyclopedia of aging.* New York: Springer Publishing Co.

Brody, H., & Vijayashanka, N. (1977). Anatomical changes in the nervous system. In C. E. Finch, & L. Hayflick (Eds.), *Handbook of the biology of aging,* New York: Van Nostrand Reinhold.

Brody, S. T., & Ruff, G. E. (Eds.). (1986). *Aging and rehabilitation.* New York: Springer Publishing Co.

Brown, J. H., Henteleff, P., Barakat, S., & Rowe, C. H. (1986). Is it normal for terminally ill patients to desire death? *American Journal of Psychiatry, 143,* 208–211.

Brown, J. H., & Paraskevas, F. (1982). Cancer and depression: Cancer presenting with depressive illness: An autoimmune disease? *British Journal of Psychiatry, 141,* 227–232.

Brown, W. T. (1987). Progeroid syndromes. In G. L. Maddox (Ed.), *The encyclopedia of aging.* New York: Springer Publishing Co.

Bryan, R. N. (1985). Imaging techniques of the aging brain. In C. M. Gaitz, & T. Samorajski (Eds.), *Aging 2000: Our health care destiny. Biomedical issues* (Vol. I). New York: Springer-Verlag.

Bullough, V., Bullough, B., & Mauro, M. (1978). Age and achievement: A dissenting view. *The Gerontologist, 18* (6), 584–587.

Burke, W. J., Rubin, E. H., Zorumski, C. F., & Wetzel, R. D. (1987). The safety of ECT in geriatric psychiatry. *Journal of the American Geriatrics Society, 35* (6), 516–521.

Burnet, F. M. (1970). An immunologic approach to aging. *Lancet, 2,* 358.

Burrus-Bammel, L. L., & Bammel, G. (1985). Leisure and recreation. In J. E. Birren, & K. W. Schaie (Eds.), *Handbook of the psychology of aging* (2nd ed.). New York: Van Nostrand Reinhold.

Busse, E. W. (1978a). Aging research: A review and critique. In G. Usdin, & C. K. Hofling (Eds.), *Aging: The process and the people.* New York: Brunner/Mazel Publishers.

Busse, E. W. (1978b). Duke longitudinal study I: Senescence and senility. In R. Katzman, R. D. Terry, & K. L. Bick (Eds.), *Alzheimer's disease: Senile dementia and related disorders (Aging,* Vol. 7). New York: Raven Press.

Busse, E. W., & Blazer, D. (1980a). Disorders related to biological functioning. In E. W. Busse & D. B. Blazer (Eds.), *Iandbook of geriatric psychiatry.* New York: Van Nostrand Reinhold.

Busse, E. W., & Blazer, D. G. (1980b). *Handbook of geriatric psychiatry.* New York: Van Nostrand Reinhold.

Busse, E. W., & Blazer, D. B. (1980c). The theories and processes of aging. In E. W. Busse, & D. G. Blazer (Eds.), *Handbook of geriatric psychiatry.* New York: Van Nostrand Reinhold.

Butler, R. N. (1963). The life review: An interpretation of reminiscence in the aged. *Psychiatry, 26,* 65–76.

Butler, R. N. (1967). The destiny of creativity in later life: Studies of creative people and the creative process. In S. Levin, & R. I. Kahana (Eds.), *Psychodynamic studies on aging: Creativity, reminiscing, and dying.* New York: International Universities Press.

Butler, R. N. (1975). Sex after 65. In L. E. Brown, & E. O. Ellis (Eds.), *Quality of life: The later years.* Acton, MA: Publishing Sciences Group.

Butler, R. N., & Lewis, M. I. (1977). *Aging and mental health: Positive psychosocial approaches.* St. Louis: C. V. Mosby Co.

Caine, E. D. (1981). Pseudodementia: Current concepts and future directions. *Archives of General Psychiatry, 38,* 1359–1364.

Calabrese, J. R., Kling, M. A., & Gold, P. W. (1987). Alterations in immunocompetence during stress, bereavement, and depression: Focus on neuroendocrine regulation. *The American Journal of Psychiatry, 144,* 1123–1134.

Campbell, J. (Ed.). (1972). *The portable Jung.* New York: The Viking Press.

Cancro, R. (1982). Schizophrenic and paranoid disorders. In D. Oken, & M. Lakovics (Eds.), *A clinical manual of psychiatry.* New York: Elsevier/North-Holland.

Cancro, R. (1985a). Overview of affective disorders. In H. I. Kaplan, & B. J. Sadock (Eds.), *Comprehensive textbook of psychiatry/IV* (Vol. 1). Baltimore, MD: Williams & Wilkins.

Cancro, R. (1985b). Schizophrenic disorders. In H. I. Kaplan, & B. J. Sadock (Eds.), *Comprehensive textbook of psychiatry/IV* (Vol. 1). Baltimore, MD: Williams & Wilkins.

Carlsson, A. (1985a). Brain neurotransmitters in normal aging. In C. M. Gaitz, & T. Samorajski (Eds.), *Aging 2000: Our health care destiny. Biomedical issues* (Vol. I). New York: Springer-Verlag.

Carlsson, A. (1985b). Neurotransmitter changes in the aging brain. *Danish Medical Bulletin, 32* (Suppl. No. 1), 40–43.

Cath, S. H. (1966). Beyond depression—The depleted state; A study in ego psychology in the aged. *Canadian Psychiatric Association Journal, 11* (Suppl.), 329–339.

Chesebro, B., Race, R., Wehrly, K., Nishio, J., et al. (1985). Identification of scrapie prion protein-specific mRNA in scrapie-infected and uninfected brain. *Nature, 315,* 331–333.

Chichester, F. C. (1968). *Gypsy moth circles the world.* New York: Coward-McCann.

Chinen, A. B. (1987). Fairy tales and psychological development in late life: A cross-cultural hermeneutic study. *The Gerontologist, 27* (3), 340–346.

Christie, A. (1960). *Murder on the Orient Express.* New York: Pocket Books.

Ciompi, L., & Müller, C. (1976). *Lebensweg und Alter der Schizophrene.* New York: Springer-Verlag.

Clark, J. E., Lanphear, A. K., & Riddick, C. C. (1987). The effects of videogame playing on the response selection processing of elderly adults. *Journal of Gerontology, 42* (1), 82–85.

Clark, R. W. (1976). *The life of Bertrand Russell.* New York: Alfred A. Knopf.

Clay, H. M. (1956). A study of performance in relation to age at two printing works. *Journal of Gerontology, 11,* 417–424.

Clayton, P. J., & Martin, R. (1980). Classification of late life organic states and the DSM-III. In N. E. Miller, & G. D. Cohen (Eds.), *Clinical aspects of Alzheimer's disease and senile dementia (Aging,* Vol. 15). New York: Raven Press.

Cohen, B. J., Cutler, R. G., & Roth, G. S. (1987). Accelerated wound repair in older mice (*Peromyscus maniculatus*) and white-footed mice (*Peromyscus leucopus*). *Journal of Gerontology, 42* (3), 302–307.

Cohen, G. D. (1977). Approach to the geriatric patient. *Medical Clinics of North America, 61*, 855–866.

Cohen, G. D. (1979). Research on aging: A piece of the puzzle. *The Gerontologist, 19*, 503–508.

Cohen, G. D. (1981). Perspectives on psychotherapy with the elderly. *American Journal of Psychiatry, 138*, 347–350.

Cohen, G. D. (1984). Practical geriatrics: The mental health professional and the Alzheimer patient. *Hospital and Community Psychiatry, 35*, 425–428.

Cohen, G. D. (1985a). The future of psychotherapy and the elderly. In C. M. Gaitz, & T. Samorajski (Eds.), *Aging 2000: Our health care destiny: Biomedical issues* (Vol. 1). New York, Springer-Verlag.

Cohen, G. D. (1985b). Toward an interface of mental and physical health phenomena in geriatrics: Clinical findings and questions. In C. M. Gaitz, & T. Samorajski (Eds.), *Aging 2000: Our health care destiny: Biomedical issues* (Vol. 1). New York, Springer-Verlag.

Cohen, D., & Eisdorfer, C. (1985). Major psychiatric and behavioral disorders in the aged. In R. Andres, E. L. Bierman, & W. R. Hazzard (Eds.), *Principles of geriatric medicine.* New York: McGraw-Hill Book Co.

Cohen, D., & Eisdorfer, C. (1986). *Loss of self: A family resource for the care of Alzheimer's disease and related disorders.* New York: W. W. Norton Company.

Colarusso, C. A., & Nemiroff, R. A. (1981). *Adult development.* New York: Plenum Press.

Cole, J. O., & Davis, J. M. (1975). Antidepressant drugs. In H. I. Kaplan, & B. J. Sadock (Eds.), *Comprehensive textbook of psychiatry/II* (Vol. I). Baltimore, MD: Williams & Wilkins.

Cole, S. (1979). Age and scientific performance. *American Journal of Sociology, 84* (4), 958–977.

Comfort, A. (1979). *The biology of senescence* (3rd ed.). London: Churchill Livingstone.

Comfort, A. (1980). Sexuality in later life. In J. E. Birren, & R. B. Sloane (Eds.), *Handbook of mental health and aging.* Englewood Cliffs, NJ: Prentice-Hall.

Cooper, A. F., Kay, D. W. K., Curry, A. R., Garside, R. F., & Roth, M. (1974). Hearing loss in paranoid and affective psychoses of the elderly. *Lancet, ii,* 851–861.

Corkin, S., Growdon, J. H., & Rasmussen, S. L. (1983). Parental age as a risk factor in Alzheimer's disease. *Annals of Neurology, 13*, 674–676.

Costa, P. T., Jr., Zonderman, A. B., McCrae, R. R., Cornoni-Huntley, Locke, B. Z., & Barbano, H. E. (1987). Longitudinal analysis of psychological well-being in a national sample: Stability of mean levels. *Journal of Gerontology, 42* (1), 50–55.

Cotman, C. W., & Holets, V. R. (1985). Structural changes at synapses with age: Plasticity and regeneration. In. C. E. Finch, & E. L. Schneider (Eds.), *Handbook of the biology of aging.* (2nd ed.). New York: Van Nostrand Reinhold.

Cotman, C. W., & Nieto-Sampedro, M. (1984). Cell biology of synaptic plasticity. *Science, 225,* 1287–1294.

Craik, F. I. M. (1984). Age differences in remembering. In L. R. Squire, & N. Butters (Eds.), *Neuropsychology of memory.* New York: The Guilford Press.

Crook, T., Bartus, R. T., Ferris, S. H., Whitehouse, P., Cohen, G. D., & Gershon, S. (1986). Age-associated memory impairment: Proposed diagnostic criteria and measures of clinical change—report of a National Institute of Mental Health work group. *Developmental Neuropsychology, 2* (4), 261–276.

Crook, T., & Cohen, G. D. (Eds.). (1981). *Physician's handbook on psychotherapeutic drug use in the aged.* New Canaan, Connecticut: Mark Powley Associates.

Cumming, E., & Henry, W. (1961). *Growing old: The process of disengagement.* New York: Basic Books.

Cutler, C. L. (1978). *How we made it to 100: Wisdom from the super old.* Rockfall, Connecticut: Rockfall Press.

Davidson, J. M. (1985). Sexuality and aging. In R. Andres, E. L. Bierman, & W. R. Hazzard (Eds.), *Principles of geriatric medicine.* New York: McGraw-Hill Book Company.

Davies, P. (1983). Neurotransmitters and neuropeptides in Alzheimer's disease. In R. Katzman (Ed.), *Biological aspects of Alzheimer's disease* (Banbury Report 15). Cold Spring Harbor, New York: Cold Spring Harbor Laboratory.

Davies, P. (1986). The genetics of Alzheimer's disease: A review and a discussion of the implications. *Neurobiology of Aging, 7,* 459–466.

Davis, J. M. (1981). Antipsychotic drugs. In T. Crook, & G. D. Cohen (Eds.), *Physician's handbook on psychotherapeutic drug use in the aged.* New Canaan, Connecticut: Mark Powley Associates.

Davis, J. M. (1985). Antipsychotic drugs. In H. I. Kaplan, & B. J. Sadock (Eds.), *Comprehensive textbook of psychiatry/IV* (Vol. II). Baltimore, MD: Williams & Wilkins.

Davison, W. (1978). The hazards of drug treatment in old age. In J. C. Brocklehurst (Ed.), *Textbook of geriatric medicine and gerontology* (2nd ed.). New York: Churchill Livingstone.

de Beauvoir, S. (1978). *The coming of age.* New York: Warner Books.

de Leon, M. J., Ferris, S. H., & George, A. E. (1985). Computerized tomography (CT) and positron emission tomography (PET) in normal and pathologic aging. In C. M. Gaitz, & T. Samorajski (Eds.), *Aging 2000: Our health care destiny* (Biomedical issues, Vol. I). New York: Springer-Verlag.

de Leon, M. J., George, A. E., & Ferris, S. H. (1986). Computed tomography and positron emission tomography correlates of cognitive decline in aging and senile dementia. In L. W. Poon (Ed.), *Handbook for clinical memory assessment of older adults.* Washington, DC: American Psychological Association.

Dennis, W. (1966). Creative productivity of persons engaged in scholarship, the sciences, and the arts. *Journal of Gerontology, 21,* 1–8.

The Diagram Group. (1983). *The brain: A users manual.* New York: A Berkley Book.

Diamond, M. C. (1983). The aging rat forebrain: Male-female left-right; Environment and lipofuscin. In D. Samuel, S. Algeri, S. Gershon, V. E. Grimm, & G. Toffan (Eds.), *Aging of the brain* (Aging, Vol. 22). New York: Raven Press.

Diamond, M. C., Krech, S., & Rosenzweig, M. R. (1964). The effects of an enriched environment on the histology of the rat cerebral cortex. *Journal of Comparative Neurology, 123,* 111–120.

Dickens, C. (1984). *A Christmas carol.* New York: A Signet Classic.

DiGiacomo, J. & Prien, R. (1983). Pharmacologic treatment of depression in the elderly. In T. Crook, & G. D. Cohen (Eds.), *Physicians' guide to the diagnosis and treatment of depression in the elderly.* New Canaan, Connecticut: Mark Powley Associates.

Drachman, D. A., & Leavitt, J. (1974). Human memory and the cholinergic system. A relationship to aging? *Archives of Neurology, 30,* 113–121.

Duffy, P., Wolf, J., Collins, G., et al. Possible person-to-person transmission of Creutzfeld-Jakob disease. *New England Journal of Medicine, 299,* 692–693.

Dyer, S., & Spragens, J. (Eds.). (1985). Diagnostic imaging: Seeing the body. In *Passages* (Vol. 1, No. 1). Washington, DC: Providence Health Foundation.

Edel, L. (1979). Portrait of the artist as an old man. In D. D. Van Tassel (Ed.), *Aging, death, and the completion of being.* Philadelphia: University of Pennsylvania Press.

Eisdorfer, C., Cohen, D., & Preston, C. (1981). Behavioral and psychological therapies for the older person with cognitive impairment. In N. E. Miller, & G. D. Cohen (Eds.), *Clinical aspects of Alzheimer's disease and senile dementia.* New York: Raven Press.

Ekerdt, D. J. (1987). Retirement. In G. L. Maddox (Ed.), *The encyclopedia of aging.* New York: Springer Publishing Co.

Epstein, C. J. (1983). Down's syndrome and Alzheimer's disease: Implications and approaches. In R. Katzman (Ed.), *Biological aspects of Alzheimer's disease* (Banbury Report 15). Cold Spring Harbor, New York: Cold Spring Harbor Laboratory.

Erikson, E. H. (1963). *Childhood and society.* New York: W. W. Norton & Company.

Estes, C. L. (1988). Cost containment and the elderly: Conflict or challenge? *Journal of the American Geriatrics Society, 36,* 68–72.

Evans, N. J. R., Baldwin, J. A., & Gath, D. (1974). The incidence of cancer among in-patients with affective disorders. *British Journal of Psychiatry, 124,* 518–525.

Exton-Smith, A. N., & Overstall. (1979). *Geriatrics.* Baltimore, MD: University Park Press.

The Federal Council on Aging. (1980). *The need for long term care* (Publication No. HHS-393). Washington, DC: U. S. Department of Health & Human Services.

Feinberg, I. (1968). The ontogenesis of human sleep and the relationship of sleep variables to intellectual function in the aged. *Comprehensive Psychiatry, 9,* 138–147.

Fernandes, G., Yunis, E. J., Jose, D. G., & Good, R. A. (1973). Dietary influence on antinuclear antibodies and cell-mediated immunity in NZB mice. *International Archives of Allergy and Applied Immunology, 44,* 770–782.

Fillit, H. M., Kemeny, E., Luine, V., Weksler, M. E., & Zabriskie, J. B. (1987). Antivascular antibodies in the sera of patients with senile dementia of the Alzheimer's type. *Journal of Gerontology, 42* (2), 180–184.

Finch, C. E. (1985a). A progress report on neurochemical and neuroendocrine regulation in normal and pathologic aging. In C. M. Gaitz, & T. Samorajski (Eds.), *Aging 2000: Our health care destiny (Biomedical issues,* Vol. I). New York: Springer-Verlag.

Finch, C. E. (1985b). Comments on review by Gash et al; Applications of recombinant DNA techniques. *Neurobiology of Aging, 6,* 156–157.

Finch, C. E. (1988). Neural and endocrine approaches to the resolution of time as a dependent variable in the aging process of mammals. *The Gerontologist, 28,* 29–42.

Finch, C. E., & Schneider, E. L. (Eds.). (1985). *Handbook of the biology of aging* (2nd ed.). New York: Van Nostrand Reinhold.

Folstein, M., Folstein, S., & McHugh, P. R. (1975). Mini-mental state: A practical method for grading the cognitive state of patients for the clinician. *Journal of Psychiatric Research, 12,* 189–198.

Folstein, M. F., Maiberger, R. & McHugh, P. R. (1977). Mood disorder as a specific complication of stroke. *Journal of Neurology, Neurosurgery, and Psychiatry, 40,* 1018–1020.

Foy, J. L. (1979). *Creative psychiatry.* New York: GEIGY Pharmaceuticals.

Frackowiak, R. S. J., & Gibbs, J. M. (1983). The pathophysiology of Alzheimer's disease studied with positron emission tomography. In R. Katzman (Ed.), *Biological aspects of Alzheimer's disease* (Banbury Report 15). Cold Spring Harbor, NY: Cold Spring Harbor Laboratory.

Franzen, M. D., & Sullivan, C. R. (1987). Cognitive rehabilitation of patients with neuropsychiatric disabilities. In R. E. Hales, & S. C. Yudofsky (Eds.), *Textbook of neuropsychiatry.* Washington, DC: American Psychiatric Press, Inc.

Freed, W. J., de Medinaceli, L., & Wyatt, R. J. (1985). Promoting functional plasticity in the damaged nervous system. *Science, 227,* 1544–1552.

Freed, W. J., Morihisa, J. M., Spoor, E., Hoffer, B. J., Olson, L., Seiger, Å., & Wyatt, R. J. (1981). Transplanted adrenal chromaffin cells in rat brain reduce lesion-induced rotational behavior. *Nature, 292,* 351–352.

Freed, W. J., Perlow, M. J., Karoum, F., Seiger, Å., Olson, L., Hoffer, B. J., & Wyatt, R. J. (1980). Restoration of dopaminergic function by grafting of fetal rat substantia nigra to the caudate nucleus: Long-term behavioral, biochemical, and histochemical studies. *Annals of Neurology, 8,* 510–519.

Freeman, E. (1978). The respiratory system. In J. C. Brocklehurst (Ed.), *Textbook of geriatric medicine and gerontology.* New York: Churchill Livingstone.

Freeman, J. T. (1979). *Aging: Its history and literature.* New York: Human Sciences Press.

Freud, S. (1978). On psychotherapy (1905). In J. Strachey (Ed. and trans.), *Complete psychological works* (Vol. 7). London: Hogarth Press.

Funkenstein, H. H., Hicks, R., Dysken, M. W., & Davis, J. M. (1981). Drug treatment of cognitive impairment in Alzheimer's disease and late life dementias. In N. E. Miller, & G. D. Cohen (Eds.), *Clinical aspects of Alzheimer's disease and senile dementia (Aging,* Vol. 5). New York: Raven Press.

Fuster, J. M. (1984). The cortical substrate of memory. In L. R. Squire, & N. Butters (Eds.), *Neuropsychology of memory.* New York: The Guilford Press.

Gaitz, C. M., & Samorajski, T. (Eds.). (1985). *Aging 2000: Our health care destiny, (Volume I: Biomedical issues.)* New York: Springer-Verlag.

Gallager, D. (1987). Caregivers of chronically ill elders. In G. G. Maddox (Ed.), *The encyclopedia of aging.* New York: Springer Publishing Co.

Gallagher, D., & Thompson, L. (1983). Effectiveness of psychotherapy for both endogenous and nonendogenous depression in older adult outpatients. *Journal of Gerontology, 38,* 707–712.

Gardner, H. (1983). *Frames of mind.* New York: Basic Books.

Garraty, J. A., & Gay, P. (Eds.). (1972). *Columbia history of the world.* New York: Harper & Row, Publishers.

Gash, D. M., Collier, T. J., & Sladek, J. R., Jr. (1985). Neural transplanation: A review of recent developments and potential applications to the aging brain. *Neurobiology of Aging, 6* (2), 131–174.

Gatz, M., Popkin, S. J., Pino, C. D., & VandenBos, G. R. (1985). Psychological interventions with older adults. In J. E. Birren, & K. W. Schaie (Eds.), *Handbook of the psychology of aging.* New York: Van Nostrand Reinhold.

Gelfand, R. (1980). Glossary. In H. I. Kaplan, A. M. Freedman, & B. J. Sadock (Eds.), *Comprehensive textbook of psychiatry/III* (Vol. 3). Baltimore, MD: Williams & Wilkins.

Gibbs, C. J., & Gajdusek, D. C. (1978). Subacute spongiform virus encephalopathies: The transmissible virus dementias. In R. Katzman, R. D. Terry, and K. L. Bick (Eds.), *Alzheimer's disease: Senile dementia and related disorders.* New York: Raven Press.

Goodnick, P. J., & Gershon, S. (1983). Chemotherapy of cognitive disorders. In D. Samuel, S. Algeri, S. Gershon, V. E. Grimm, & G. Toffano (Eds.), *Aging of the brain.* New York: Raven Press.

Goodnick, P., Gershon, S., & Salzman, C. (1984). Evaluation and management of dementia. In C. Salzman (Ed.), *Clinical geriatric psychopharmacology.* New York: McGraw-Hill.

Granick, S. (1971). Psychological test functioning. In S. Granick & R. Patterson (Eds.), *Human aging II: An eleven-year followup biomedical and behavioral study* (DHEW Publication No. (HSM) 71-9037). Washington, DC: U. S. Government Printing Office.

Granick, S., & Patterson, R. D. (Eds.). (1971). *Human aging II: An eleven-year followup biomedical and behavioral study* (DHEW Publication No. (HSM) 71-9037). Washington, DC: U. S. Government Printing Office.

Grotjahn, M. (1955). Analytic psychotherapy with the elderly, I: The sociological background of aging in America. *Psychoanalitic Review, 42,* 419–427.

Gruman, G. J. (1966). A history of ideas about the prolongation of life: The evolution of prolongevity hypotheses to 1800. *Transactions of the American Philosophical Society, 56* (9), 1–102.

Guillerme, J. (1963). *Longevity.* New York: Walker and Co.

Gustafson, L. (1985). Differential diagnosis with special reference to treatable dementias and pseudodementia conditions. *Danish Medical Bulletin, 32* (Supplement 1), 55–60.

Habot, B., & Libow, L. L. (1980). The interrelationship of mental and physical status and its assessment in the older adult: Mind-body interaction. In J. E. Birren, & R. B. Sloane (Eds.), *Handbook of mental health and aging.* Englewood Cliffs, NJ: Prentice-Hall.

Hachinski, V. C. (1983). Differential diagnosis of Alzheimer's disease: Multi-infarct dementia. In B. Reisberg (Ed.), *Alzheimer's disease.* New York: The Free Press.

Hachinski, V. C., Iliff, L. E., Zilhka, E., et al. (1975). Cerebral blood flow in dementia. *Archives of Neurology, 32,* 632–637.

Hagestad, G. O., & Neugarten, B. L. (1985). Age and the life course. In R. B. Binstock, & E. Shanus (Eds.), *Handbook of aging and the social sciences* (2nd Ed.). New York: Van Nostrand Reinhold.

Haley, W. E., Levine, E. G., Brown, S. L., Berry, J. W., & Hughes, G. H. (1987). Psychological, social, and health consequences of caring for a relative with senile dementia. *Journal of the American Geriatrics Society, 35,* 405–411.

Harris, L., & Associates. (1975). *The myth and reality of aging in America.* Washington, DC: The National Council on the aging.

Harrison, T. R., et al. (Eds.). (1966). *Principles of internal medicine* (5th ed.). New York: McGraw-Hill.

Hartford, J. T., & Samorajski, T. (Eds.). (1984). *Alcoholism in the elderly: Social and biomedical issues.* New York: Raven Press.

Haug, H. (1985). Are neurons of the human cerebral cortex really lost during aging? A morphologic examination. In J. Traber, & W. H. Gispen (Eds.), *Senile dementia of the Alzheimer type.* Berlin: Springer-Verlag.

Hayflick, L. (1977). The cellular basis for biological aging. In C. E. Finch, & L. Hayflick (Eds.), *Handbook of the biology of aging* (1st ed.). New York: Van Nostrand Reinhold.

Hayflick, L. (1985). Theories of biological aging. In R. Andres, E. L. Bierman, & W. R. Hazzard (Eds.), *Principles of geriatric medicine.* New York: McGraw-Hill.

Hayflick, L. (1987a). Biological theories of aging. In G. L. Maddox (Ed.), *The encyclopedia of aging.* New York: Springer Publishing Co.

Hayflick, L. (1987b). Cell aging *in vivo.* In G. L. Maddox (Ed.), *The encyclopedia of aging.* New York: Springer Publishing Co.

Hearn, H. L. (1972). Aging and the artistic career. *The Gerontologist, Winter,* 357–362.

Hemingway, E. (1980). *The old man and the sea.* New York: Charles Scribner's Sons.

Hendin, H. (1982). *Suicide in America.* New York: W. W. Norton and Company.

Hendricks, J., & Hendricks. (1977). *Aging in mass society: Myths and realities.* Cambridge, MA: Winthrop Publishers.

Heston, L. L. (1983). Dementia of the Alzheimer type: A perspective from family studies. In R. Katzman (Ed.), *Biological aspects of Alzheimer's disease* (Banbury Report 15). Cold Spring Harbor, NY: Cold Spring Harbor Laboratory.

Heston, L. L., & White, J. A. (1983). *Dementia—a practical guide to Alzheimer's disease and related disorders.* New York: W. H. Freeman and Company.

Holliday, R., Hutschtscha, L. I., Tarran, G. M., & Kirkwood, T. B. L. (1977). Testing the commitment theory of cellular aging. *Science, 190,* 136–137.

Hollister, L. E. (1981). General principles of psychotherapeutic drug use in the aged. In T. Crook, & G. D. Cohen (Eds.), *Physician's handbook on psychotherapeutic drug use in the aged.* New Canaan, CT: Mark Powley Associates.

Holzer, C. E., Robins, L. N., Myers, J. K., Weismann, M. M., Tischler, G. L., Leaf, P. J., Anthony, J., & Bednarski, P. B. (1984). Antecedents and correlates of alcohol abuse and dependence in the elderly. In G. Maddox, L. N. Robins, & N. Rosenberg (Eds). *Nature and extent of alcohol problems among the elderly.* Rockville, MD: Alcohol, Drug Abuse, and Mental Health Administration DHHS Publication No. (ADM) 84-1321.

Huang, L., Cartwright, W. S., & Hu, T. (1988). The economic cost of senile dementia in the United States. *Public Health Reports, 103,* 3–7.

Hyman, B. T., Van Hoesen, G. W., Damasio, A. R., & Barnes, C. L. (1984). Alzheimer's disease: Cell-specific pathology isolates the hippocampal formation. *Science, 225,* 1168–1170.

Iqbal, K., Grundke-Iqbal, I., Wisniewski, H. M., & Terry, R. D. (1978). Neurofibers in Alzheimer dementia and other conditions. In R. Katzman, R. D. Terry, & K. L. Bick (Eds.), *Alzheimer's disease: Senile dementia and related disorders* (*Aging,* Vol. 7). New York: Raven Press.

Jacobs, S., & Ostfeld, A. (1977). An epidemiological review of the mortality of bereavement. *Psychosomatic Medicine, 39,* 344–357.

Jaffe, A. J. (1972). The retirement dilemma. *Journal of Industrial Gerontology, 14,* 1–89.

Jarvik, L., & Falek, A. (1963). Intellectual ability and survival in the aged. *Journal of Gerontology, 18,* 173–176.

Jarvik, L., & Greenson H. (Transls). (1987). About a peculiar disease of the cerebral cortex by Alois Alzheimer. *Alzheimer's Disease and Associated Disorders, 1* (1), 7–8.

Jarvik, L. F., & Perl, M. (1981). Overview of physiologic dysfunctions related to psychiatric problems in the elderly. In A. J. Levenson, & R. C. W. Hall (Eds.), *Neuropsychiatric manifestations of physical disease in the elderly.* New York: Raven Press.

Johnson, R. T., (1982). *Viral infections of the nervous system.* New York: Raven Press.

Jones, E. (1957). *The life and work of Sigmund Freud* (Vol. 3). New York: Basic Books.

Kahn, R. L., Goldfarb, A. I., Pollack, M., & Peck, A. (1960). Brief objective measures for the determination of mental status of the aged. *American Journal of Psychiatry, 117,* 326–328.

Kahn, R. L., & Tobin, S. S. (1981). Community treatment for aged persons with altered brain function. In N. E. Miller, & G. D. Cohen (Eds.), *Clinical aspects of Alzheimer's disease and senile dementia* (pp. 253–276). New York: Raven Press.

Kahn, R. L., Zarit, S., Hilbert, N. M., & Niederehe, G. (1975). Memory complaint and impairment in the aged. *Archives of General Psychiatry, 32,* 1569–1573.

Kalish, R. A. (1976). Death and dying in a social context. In R. H. Binstock, & E. Shanus (Eds.), *Handbook of aging and the social sciences.* New York: Van Nostrand Reinhold.

Kandel, E. R. (1983). From metapsychology to molecular biology: Explorations into the nature of anxiety. *American Journal of Psychiatry, 140,* 1277–1293.

Kaplan, H. I., & Sadock, B. J. (1980). Neurophysiology of behavior. In H. I. Kaplan, A. M. Freedman, & B. J. Sadock (Eds.), *Comprehensive textbook of psychiatry/III* (Vol. 1). Baltimore, MD: Williams & Wilkins.

Kaplan, H. I., & Sadock, B. J. (Eds.). (1985). *Comprehensive textbook of psychiatry/IV.* Baltimore, MD: Williams & Wilkins.

Karasu, T. B. (Ed.). (1984). *The psychiatric therapies.* Washington, DC: American Psychiatric Association.

Karlsson, J. L. (1970). Genetic association of giftedness and creativity with schizophrenia. *Hereditas, 66,* 177.

Kastenbaum, R. (1985). Dying and death: A life-span approach. In J. E. Birren, & K. W. Schaie (Eds.), *Handbook of the psychology of aging* (2nd ed.). New York: Van Nostrand Reinhold.

Katz, S. E. (1985). Psychiatric hospitalization. In H. I. Kaplan, & B. J. Sadock (Eds.), *Comprehensive textbook of psychiatry/IV* (Vol. II). Baltimore, MD: Williams & Wilkins.

Katzman, R. (Ed.). (1983). *Biological aspects of Alzheimer's disease* (Banbury Report 15). Cold Spring Harbor, NY: Cold Spring Harbor Laboratory.

Katzman, R. (1986). Medical progress: Alzheimer's disease. *New England Journal of Medicine, 314,* 964–973.

Katzman, R., Terry, R. D., & Bick, K. L. (Eds.). (1976). *Alzheimer's Disease: Senile dementia and related disorders.* New York: Raven Press.

Kelleher, C. H., & Quirk, D. A. (1973). Age, functional capacity, and work: An annotated bibliography. *Industrial Gerontology, 19,* 80–98.

Kendig, F., & Hutton, R. (1979). *Life spans or how long things last.* New York: Holt, Rinehart and Winston.

Kirkwood, T. B. L. (1985). Comparative and evolutionary aspects of longevity. In C. E. Finch, & E. L. Schneider (Eds.), *Handbook of the biology of aging* (2nd ed.). New York: Van Nostrand Reinhold.

Klerman, G. L. (1982). Affective disorders: Depressions and mania. In D. Oken, & M. Lakovics (Eds.), *A clinical manual of psychiatry.* New York: Elsevier/ North-Holland.

Kogan, N. (1975). Creativity and cognitive style. In P. B. Baltes, & K. W. Schaie (Eds.), *Lifespan developmental psychology: Personality and socialization.* New York: Academic Press.

Kohn, R. R. (1971). Effect of antioxidants on life-span of C57BL mice. *Journal of Gerontology, 26,* 378–380.

Kordower, J. H. R. L., Dean, H. C., White, F., & Marciano, F. F. (1988). Transplantation into the mammalian CNS: A meeting report on the sixth Schmitt neurological sciences symposium. *Neurobiology Of Aging, 9,* 127–137.

Kosei, O., & Appel, S. H. (1983). Neurotrophic factors and Alzheimer's disease. In R. Katzman (Ed.), *Biological aspects of Alzheimer's disease* (Banbury Report 15). Cold Spring Harbor, NY: Cold Spring Harbor Laboratory.

Kral, V. A. (1978). Benign senescent forgetfulness. In R. Katzman, R. D. Terry, & K. L. Bick (Eds.), *Alzheimer's disease: Senile dementia and related disorders (Aging,* Vol. 7). New York: Raven Press.

Kuhl, D. E., Metter, E. J., Riege, W. H., & Hawkins, R. A. (1985). Determination of cerebral glucose utilization in dementia using positron emission tomography. *Danish Medical Bulletin, 32* (Supplement 1), 51–55.

Lamy, P. P. (1980). *Prescribing for the elderly.* Littleton, MA: PSG Medical Books.

Larson, E. B., Buchner, D. M., Uhlmann, R. F., & Reifler, B. V. (1986). Caring for elderly patients with dementia. *Archives of International Medicine, 146,* 1909–1910.

LaRue, A., Dessonville, C., & Jarvik, L. F. (1985). Aging and mental disorders. In J. E. Birren, & K. W. Schaie (Eds.), *Handbook of the psychology of aging.* New York: Van Nostrand Reinhold.

Lauter, H. (1985). What do we know about Alzheimer's disease today? *Danish Medical Bulletin, 32* (Supplement 1), 1–21.

Lawton, M. P. (1981). Sensory deprivation and the effect of the environment on management of the patient with senile dementia. In N. E. Miller, & G. D. Cohen (Eds.), *Clinical aspects of Alzheimer's disease and senile dementia.* New York: Raven Press.

Lehman, H. C. (1953). *Age and achievement.* Princeton, NJ: Princeton University Press.

Levenson, A. J. (Ed.). (1979). *Neuropsychiatric side effects of drugs in the elderly.* New York: Raven Press.

Levitan, S. T., & Kornfeld, D. S. (1981). Clinical and cost benefits of liaison psychiatry. *American Journal of Psychiatry, 138,* 790–793.

Lewin, R. (1987). Dramatic results with brain grafts. *Science, 237,* 245–247.

Lieberman, L., & Lieberman, L. (1983). Second careers in art and craft fairs. *The Gerontologist, 23* (3), 266–272.

Lipowski, Z. J. (1980). Organic mental disorders: Introduction and review of syndromes. In H. I. Kaplan, A. M. Freedman, & B. J. Sadock (Eds.), *Comprehensive textbook of psychiatry* (Vol. 2). Baltimore, MD: Williams & Wilkins.

Lipowski, Z. J. (1981). Organic mental disorders: Their history and classification with special reference to DSM-III. In N. E. Miller, & G. D. Cohen, *Clinical aspects of Alzheimer's disease and senile dementia (Aging,* Vol. 15). New York: Raven Press.

Lipowski, Z. J. (1983). Transient cognitive disorders (delirium, acute confusional states) in the elderly. *American Journal of Psychiatry, 140* (11), 1426–1436.

Mace, N. L., & Rabins, P. V. (1981). *The 36-hour day.* Baltimore, MD: The Johns Hopkins University Press.

Maddox, G., Robins, L. N., & Rosenberg, N. (Eds.). (1984). *Nature and extent of alcohol problems among the elderly.* Rockville, MD: Alcohol, Drug Abuse, and Mental Health Administration DHHS Publication No. (ADM) 84-1321.

Madrazo, I., Drucker-Colin, R., Díaz, V., Martínez-Mata, J., Torres, C., & Becerril, J. J. (1987). Open microsurgical autograft of adrenal medulla to the right caudate nucleus in two patients with intractable Parkinson's disease. *The New England Journal of Medicine, 316* (14), 831–834.

Maduro, R. (1974). Artistic creativity and aging in India. *International Journal of Aging and Human Development, 5* (4), 303–329.

Makinodan, T. (1977). Immunity and aging. In C. E. Finch, & L. Hayflick (Eds.), *Handbook of the biology of aging* (1st ed.). New York: Van Nostrand Reinhold.

Mann, D. M. A. (1985). Commentary on review by D. M. Gash, T. J. Collier and J. R. Sladek (on) the application of neural transplantation to degenerative disease of the human nervous system. *Neurobiology of Aging, 6,* 160–162.

Manton, K. G., Blazer, D. G., & Woodbury, M. A. (1987). Suicide in middle age and later life: sex and race specific life table and cohort analysis. *Journal of Gerontology, 42* (2), 219–227.

Manuelidis, E. E., de Figueiredo, J. M., Kim, J. H., Fritch, W. W., & Manuelidis, L. (1988). Transmission studies from blood of Alzheimer disease patients and healthy relatives. *Proceedings of the National Academy of Sciences, 85,* 4898–4901.

Maslow, A. (1959). Creativity in self-actualizing people. In H. H. Anderson (Ed.), *Creativity and its cultivation.* New York: Harper & Row.

Masoro, E. J. (1987). Life extension. In G. L. Maddox (Ed.), *The encyclopedia of aging.* New York: Springer Publishing Co.

Masters, W, H., & Johnson, V. E. (1981). Sex and the aging process. *Journal of the American Geriatrics Society, 29,* 385–390.

Mayeux, R., Stern, Y., Rosen, J., & Levanthal, J. (1981). Depression, intellectual impairment, and Parkinson disease. *Neurology, 31,* 645–650.

McGrady, P. M. (1968). *The youth doctors.* New York: Coward-McCann.

McKhann, G., Drachman, D., Folstein, M., Katzman, R., Price, D., & Stadlan, E. M. (1984). Clinical diagnosis of Alzheimer's disease. *Neurology, 34,* 939–944.

McLeish, J. A. B. (1976). *The Ulyssean adult: Creativity in the middle & later years.* New York: McGraw-Hill Ryerson Limited.

McLeish, J. A. B. (1981). The continuum of creativity. In P. W. Johnston (Ed.), *Perspectives on aging: Exploding the myth.* Cambridge, MA: Ballinger Publishing Co.

Merriam, A. E., Aronson, M. K., Gaston, P., Wey, S., & Katz, I. (1988). The psychiatric symptoms of Alzheimer's disease. *Journal of the American Geriatrics Society, 36,* 7–12.

Merz, P. A., Rohwer, R. G., Kascsak, R., Wisniewski, H. M., Somerville, R. A., Gibbs, C. J., & Gajdusek, D. C. (1984). Infection-specific particle from the unconventional slow virus diseases. *Science, 225,* 437–440.

Miller, N. E., & Bartus, R. T. (1982). Sleep, sleep pathology, and psychopathology in later life: A new research frontier. *Neurobiology of Aging, 3,* 283–286.

Miller, N. E., & Cohen, G. D. (1981). *Clinical aspects of Alzheimer's disease and senile dementia* (*Aging*, Vol. 15). New York: Raven Press.

Miller, N. E., & Cohen, G. D. (1987). *Schizophrenia and aging.* New York: The Guilford Press.

Mobley, W. C., Rutkowski, J. L., Tennekoon, G. I., Buchanan, K., & Johnston, M. V. (1985). Choline acetyltransferase activity in striatum of neonatal rats increased by nerve growth factor. *Science, 229,* 284–287.

Mooradian, A. D. (1988). Effect of aging on the blood-brain barrier. *Neurobiology Of Aging, 9,* 31–39.

Morley, J. E. (1986). Neuropeptides, behavior, and aging. *Journal of the American Geriatrics Society, 34* (1), 52–62.

Mortimer, J. A., French, L. R., Hutton, J. T., and Schuman, L. M. (1985). Head injury as a risk factor for Alzheimer's disease. *Neurology (NY), 35,* 264–267.

Moss, R. J., & Miles, S. H. (1987). AIDS and the geriatrician. *Journal of the American Geriatrics Society, 35,* 460–464.

Moylan, J. A., & Flye, M. W. (1978). Peripheral vascular disease in the geriatric patient. In W. Reichel (Ed.), *Clinical aspects of aging.* Baltimore, MD: Williams & Wilkins.

Mumford, E., Schlesinger, H. J., & Glass, G. V. (1982). The effects of psychological intervention on recovery from surgery and heart attacks: An analysis of the literature. *American Journal of Public Health, 72,* 141–151.

Myers, G. C. (1987). *The encyclopedia of aging.* New York: Springer Publishing Co.

Nandy, K., & Bourne, G. H. (1966). Effect of centrophenoxine on the lipofuscin pigments in the neurones of senile guinea-pigs. *Nature, 210,* 313–314.

National Advisory Mental Health Council (1988). *Report of the National Advisory Mental Health Council on a national plan for schizophrenia research.* Washington, DC: Alcohol, Drug Abuse, and Mental Health Administration.

National Institute of Mental Health. (1981). *National Institute of Mental Health Science Reports: Special report on depression research* (DHHS Publication No. (ADM) 81-1085). Rockville, MD: National Institute of Mental Health.

National Institute on Aging Task Force. (1980). Senility reconsidered—Treatment possibilities for mental impairment of the elderly. *Journal of the American Medical Association, 244,* 259–263.

Neugarten, B. L., Moore, J. W., & Lowe, J. C. (1965). Age norms, age constraints, and adult socialization. *American Journal of Sociology, 70,* 710–717.

Newell, F. W. (1982). *Ophthalmology—Principles and concepts.* St. Louis: The C. V. Mosby Co.

Newman, G., & Nichols, C. R. (1970). Sexual activities and attitudes in older persons. In E. Palmore (Ed.), *Normal aging.* Durham, NC: Duke University Press.

Nickens, H. W., Crook, T., & Cohen, G. D. (1986). Psychotropic drugs. *Generations, 10,* 33–37.

Niemi, T., & Jaaskelainen, J. (1978). Cancer morbidity in depressed persons. *Journal of Psychosomatic Research, 22,* 117–120.

Nolan, L., & O'Malley, K. (1988a). Prescribing for the elderly, part I: Sensitivity of the elderly to adverse drug reactions. *Journal of the American Geriatrics Society, 36,* 142–149.

Nolan, L., & O'Malley, K. (1988b). Prescribing for the elderly, part II: Sensitivity of the elderly to adverse drug reactions. *Journal of the American Geriatrics Society, 36,* 245–254.

O'Casey, S. (1968). Crabbed age and youth. In B. Atkinson (Ed.), *The Sean O'Casey reader.* New York: St. Martin's Press.
Oesch, B., Westaway, D., Wälchli, et al. (1985). A cellular gene encodes scrapie PrP 27-30 protein. *Cell, 40,* 735–746.
Okun, M. A., & Elias, C. S. (1977). Cautiousness in adulthood as a function of age and payoff structure. *Journal of Gerontology, 32,* 451–455.
Owens, W. A. (1953). Age and mental abilities: A longitudinal study. *Genetic Psychology Monographs, 48,* 3–54.
Owens, W. A. (1966). Age and mental abilities: A second adult follow-up. *Journal of Educational Psychology, 57,* 311–325.
Paffenbarger, R. S., Hyde, R. T., Wing, A. L., & Steinmetz, C. H. (1984). A natural history of athleticism and cardiovascular health. *Journal of the American Medical Association, 252,* 491–495.
Palmore, E. (1979). Predictors of successful aging. *The Gerontologist, 19,* 427–431.
Palmore, E. B. (1987). Centenarians. In G. L. Maddox (Ed.), *The encyclopedia of aging.* New York: Springer Publishing Co.
Parnes, H. S., & Nestel, G. (1981). The retirement experience. In H. S. Parnes (Ed.), *Work and retirement: A longitudinal study of men.* Cambridge, MA: MIT Press.
Pearson, D., & Shaw, S. (1982). *Life extension.* New York: Warner Books.
Perl, D. P. (1983). Pathologic association of aluminum in Alzheimer's disease. In B. Reisberg (Ed.), *Alzheimer's disease: The standard reference.* New York: The Free Press.
Perlow, M. F., Freed, W. F., Hoffer, B. J., Seiger, A., Olson, L., & Wyatt, R. J., (1979). Brain grafts reduce motor abnormalities produced by destruction of nigrostriatal dopamine system. *Science, 204,* 643–647.
Perry, E. K., & Perry, R. H. (1985). A review of neuropathological and neurochemical correlates of Alzheimer's disease. *Danish Medical Bulletin, 32* (Supplement 1), 27–34.
Pert, C. B., Ruff, M. R., Weber, R. J., et al. (1985). Neuropeptides and their receptors: A psychosomatic network. *The Journal of Immunology, 135,* 820s–826s.
Pfeiffer, E. (1975). A short portable mental status questionnaire for the assessment of organic brain deficit in elderly patients. *Journal of the American Geriatrics Society, 23,* 433–441.
Pfeiffer, E. (1976). Psychotherapy with elderly patients. In L. Ballak & T. Karasu (Eds.), *Geriatric psychiatry.* New York: Grune & Stratton.
Plotkin, D. A., Mintz, J., & Jarvik, L. F. (1985). Subjective memory complaints in geriatric depression. *American Journal of Psychiatry, 142,* 1103–1105.
Polednak, A. P., & Damon, A. (1970). College athletics, longevity and cause of death. *Human Biology, 42,* 28–46.
Poon, L. W. (Ed.). (1986). *Handbook for clinical memory assessment of older adults.* Washington, DC: American Psychological Association.
Poon, L. W. (1987). Learning. In G. L. Maddox (Ed.), *The encyclopedia of aging.* New York: Springer Publishing Co.
Post, F. (1980). Paranoid, schizophrenia-like, and schizophrenic states in the aged. In J. E. Birren, & R. B. Sloane (Eds.), *Handbook of mental health and aging.* Englewood Cliffs, NJ: Prentice-Hall.
Prusiner, S. B., Bolton, D. C., Bowman, K. A., Groth, D. F., et al. (1983). Prions and dementia. In R. Katzman (Ed.), *Biological aspects of Alzheimer's disease,* (Banbury Report 15). Cold Spring Harbor, NY: Cold Spring Harbor Laboratory.

The Random House Dictionary. (1971). *The Random House dictionary of the English language.* New York: Random House.

Rechtschaffen, A. (1959). Psychotherapy with geriatric patients: A review of the literature. *Journal of Gerontology, 14,* 73–84.

Regestein, Q. R. (1984). Treatment of insomnia in the elderly. In C. Salzman (Ed.), *Clinical geriatric psychopharmacology.* New York: McGraw-Hill.

Reifler, B. V., & Larson, E. (1988). Excess disability in demented elderly outpatients: The rule of the halves. *Journal of the American Geriatrics Society, 36,* 82–83.

Reifler, B. V., Larson, E., Teri, L., & Poulsen, M. (1986). Dementia of the Alzheimer's type and depression. *Journal of the American Geriatrics Society, 34,* 855–859.

Reisberg, B. (1981). *Brain failure: An introduction to current concepts of senility.* New York: The Free Press.

Reisberg, B. (Ed.). (1983). *Alzheimer's disease.* New York: The Free Press.

Reisberg, B., & Ferris, S. H. (1982). Diagnosis and assessment of the older patient. *Hospital and Community Psychiatry, 33,* 104–110.

Reiser, M. F. (1984). *Mind, brain, body.* New York: Basic Books.

Reker, G. T., Peacock, E. J., & Wong, T. P. (1987). Meaning and purpose in life and well-being: A life-span perspective. *Journal of Gerontology, 42* (1), 44–49.

Restak, R. M. (1980). *The brain.* New York: Warner Books.

Reynolds, C. F., Kupfer, D. J., & Sewitch, D. E. (1984). Practical geriatrics: Diagnosis and management of sleep disorders in the elderly. *Hospital and Community Psychiatry, 35,* 779–781.

Riege, W. H., & Metter, E. J. (1988). Cognitive and brain imaging measures of Alzheimer's disease. *Neurobiology Of Aging, 9,* 69–86.

Riga, S., & Riga, D. (1974). Effects of centrophenoxine on the lipofuscin pigments in the nervous system of old rats. *Brain Research, 72,* 265–275.

Roberts, M. (1979). *Chinese fairy tales and fantasies.* New York: Pantheon.

Robinson, P. K., Coberly, S., & Paul, C. E. (1985). Work and retirement. In R. H. Binstock, & E. Shanus (Eds.), *Handbook of aging and the social sciences,* (2nd ed.). New York: Van Nostrand Reinhold.

Robinson, R. G., & Forrester, A. W. (1987). Neuropsychiatric aspects of cerebrovascular disease. In R. E. Hales, & S. C. Yudofsky (Eds.), *Textbook of Neuropsychiatry.* Washington, DC: The American Psychiatric Press.

Rockstein, M., Chesky, J. A., & Sussman, M. L. (1977). Comparative biology and evolution of aging. In C. E. Finch, & L. Hayflick (Eds.), *Handbook of the biology of aging,* (1st ed.) New York: Van Nostrand Reinhold.

Rodin, G., & Voshart, K. (1986). Depression in the medically ill: An overview. *American Journal of Psychiatry, 143,* 696–705.

Roosevelt, E. (1958). *On my own.* New York: Harper & Brothers Publishers.

Rosenberg, G. S., Greenwald, B., & Davis, K. L. (1983). Pharmacologic treatment of Alzheimer's disease: An overview. In B. Reisberg (Ed.), *Alzheimer's disease: The standard reference.* New York: The Free Press.

Rosse, R. B., & Morihisa, J. M. (1988). Brain imaging. In J. Talbott, R. E. Hales, & S. C. Yudofsky (Eds.), *The American psychiatric press textbook of psychiatry.* Washington, DC: American Psychiatric Press.

Rossor, M. M. (1985). Neuropeptides in human aging and dementia. In C. M. Gaitz, & T. Samorajski (Eds.), *Aging 2000: Our health care destiny. (Biomedical issues,* Vol. I). New York: Springer-Verlag.

Roth, M. (1955). The natural history of mental disorder in old age. *Journal of Mental Science, 101,* 281–301.

Roth, M. (1978). Diagnosis of senile and related forms of dementia. In R. Katzman, R. D. Terry, & K. L. Bick (Eds.), *Alzheimer's disease: Senile dementia and related disorders (Aging,* Vol. 7). New York: Raven Press.

Rowe, J. W., & Kahn, R. L. (1987). Human aging: Usual and successful. *Science, 237,* 143–149.

Ruben, R. J. (1978). Otolaryngologic problems. In W. Reichel (Ed.), *The Geriatric Patient.* New York: HP Publishing Co.

Russell, B. (1960). *Bertrand Russell speaks his mind.* New York: Bard Books. Published by Avon Book Division.

Sacher, G. A. (1977). Life table modification and life prolongation. In C. E. Finch, & L. Hayflick (Eds.), *Handbook of the biology of aging* (1st ed.). New York: Van Nostrand Reinhold.

Sadavoy, J., & Leszcz, M. (Eds.). (1987). *Treating the elderly with psychotherapy: The scope for change in later life.* Madison, CT: International Universities Press.

Sagan, C. (1977). *The dragons of Eden.* New York: Ballantine Books.

Sajdel-Sulkowska, E. M., & Marotta, C. A. (1984). Alzheimer's disease brain: Alterations in RNA levels and in a ribonuclease-inhibitor complex. *Science, 255,* 947–949.

Sakauye, K. M. (1986). Practical geriatrics: A model for administration of electroconvulsive therapy. *Hospital and Community Psychiatry, 37,* 785–788.

Salzman, C. (1982). Basic principles of psychotropic drug prescription for the elderly. *Hospital and Community Psychiatry, 33,* 133–136.

Salzman, C. (1983). Depression and physical disease. In T. Crook, & G. D. Cohen (Eds.), *Physician's guide to the diagnosis and treatment of depression in the elderly.* New Canaan, CT: Mark Powley Associates.

Salzman, C. (1984a). Neurotransmission in the aging central nervous system. In C. Salzman (Ed.), *Clinical geriatric psychopharmacology.* New York: McGraw-Hill.

Salzman, C. (1984b). Psychotropic drug dosages and drug interactions. In C. Salzman (Ed.), *Clinical geriatric psychopharmacology.* New York: McGraw-Hill.

Salzman, C. (Ed.). (1984c). *Clinical geriatric psychopharmacology.* New York: McGraw-Hill.

Sanadi, D. R. (1977). Metabolic changes and their significance in aging. In C. E. Finch, & L. Hayflick (Eds.), *Handbook of the biology of aging* (1st ed.). New York: Van Nostrand Reinhold.

Schaie, K. W. (1980). Intelligence and problem solving. In J. E. Birren, & R. B. Sloane (Eds.), *Handbook of mental health and aging.* Englewood Cliffs, NJ: Prentice-Hall.

Schaie, K. W., & Parham, I. A. (1977). Cohort-sequential analyses of adult intellectual development. *Developmental Psychology, 13,* 649–653.

Schildkraut, J. J. (1974). Biogenic amines and affective disorders. *Annual Review of Medicine, 25,* 333–348.

Schneider, E. L., & Reed, J. D. (1985). Life extension. *New England Journal of Medicine, 312,* 1159–1168.

Schneider, G. E. (1979). Is it better to have your brain lesion early? A revision of the "Kennard principle." *Neuropsychologia, 17* (6), 557–583.

Segerberg, O., Jr. (1982). *Living to be 100.* New York: Charles Scribner's Sons.

Selkoe, D. J. (1986). Altered structural proteins in plaques and tangles: What do they tell us about Alzheimer's disease? *Neurobiology of Aging, 7,* 425–432.

Selmanowitz, V. J., Rizer, R. L., & Orentreich, N. (1977). Aging of the skin and its appendages. In C. E. Finch, & L. Hayflick (Eds.), *Handbook of the biology of aging* (1st ed.). New York: Van Nostrand Reinhold.

Seneca, L. A. (1926). On old age. In L. Wann (Ed.), *Century readings in the English essay.* New York: Appleton-Century-Crofts.

Sharps, M. J., & Gollin, E. S. (1987). Speed and accuracy of mental image rotation in young and elderly adults. *Journal of Gerontology, 42* (3), 342–344.

Shavit, Y., Terman, G. W., Martin, F. C., et al. (1985). Stress, opioid peptides, the immune system, and cancer. *The Journal of Immunology, 135,* 834s–837s.

Shekelle, R. B., Raynor, W. J., Ostfeld, A. M., et al. (1981). Psychological depression and 17 year risk of death from cancer. *Psychosomatic Medicine, 43,* 117–125.

Sheldon, A., McEwan, P. J. M., & Ryser, C. P. (1975). *Retirement: Patterns and predictions* (DHEW Publication No. (ADM) 74-49). Washington, DC: U. S. Government Printing Office.

Shepherd, G. M. (1983). *Neurobiology.* New York: Oxford University Press.

Sheppard, H. L. (1976). Work and retirement. In R. H. Binstock, & E. Shanus (Eds.), *Handbook of aging and the social sciences* (1st ed.). New York: Van Nostrand Reinhold.

Shock, N. W. (1977). Systems integration. In C. E. Finch, & L. Hayflick (Eds.), *Handbook of the biology of aging* (1st ed.). New York: Van Nostrand Reinhold.

Shock, N. W., Grevlich, R. C., Andres, R., et al. (Eds.). (1984). *Normal human aging: The Baltimore longitudinal study of aging* (NIH Publication No. 84-2450). Washington, DC: U. S. Government Printing Office.

Siegler, I. C. (1980). The psychology of adult development and aging. In E. W. Busse, & D. G. Blazer (Eds.), *Handbook of geriatric psychiatry.* New York: Van Nostrand Reinhold.

Siever, L. J., & Davis, K. L. (1985). Overview: Toward a dysregulation hypothesis of depression. *American Journal of Psychiatry, 142,* 1017–1031.

Simmons, L. W. (1945). *The role of the aged in primitive society.* New Haven, CT: Yale University Press.

Simon, A. (1980). Alcoholism. In J. E. Birren, & R. B. Sloane (Eds.), *Handbook of mental health and aging.* Englewood Cliffs, NJ: Prentice-Hall.

Sklar, M. (1978). Gastrointestinal diseases in the aged. In W. Reichel (Ed.), *Clinical aspects of aging.* Baltimore, MD: Williams & Wilkins.

Sladek, J. R., & Shoulson, I. (1988). Neural transplantation: A call for patience rather than patients. *Science, 240,* 1386–1388.

Sloane, R. B. (1980). Organic brain syndrome. In J. E. Birren, & R. B. Sloane (Eds.), *Handbook of mental health and aging.* Englewood Cliffs, NJ: Prentice-Hall.

Solomon, P., & Kleeman, S. T. (1985). Sensory deprivation. In H. I. Kaplan, & B. J. Sadock (Eds.), *Comprehensive textbook of psychiatry/IV* (Vol. 1). Baltimore, MD: Williams & Wilkins.

Solomon, S. (1985). Neurological evaluation. In H. I. Kaplan, & B. J. Sadock (Eds.), *Comprehensive textbook of psychiatry/IV* (Vol. I). Baltimore, MD: Williams & Wilkins.

Sorenson, J. R. J., Campbell, I. R., Tepper, L. B., & Lingg, R. D. (1974). Aluminum in the environment and human health. *Environmental Health Perspectives, 8,* 3–95.

Squire, L. R., & Butters, N. (Eds.). (1984). *Neuropsychology of memory.* New York: The Guilford Press.

Stagner, R. (1985). Aging in industry. In J. E. Birren, & K. W. Schaie (Eds.), *Handbook of the psychology of aging* (2nd ed.). New York: Van Nostrand Reinhold.

Stedman's Medical Dictionary (21st ed.). (1966). Baltimore, MD: Williams & Wilkins.

Stein, M., Keller, S. E., & Schleifer, S. J. (1985). Stress and immunomodulation: The role of depression and neuroendocrine function. *The Journal of Immunology, 135,* 827s–833s.

St George-Hyslop, P. H., Tanzi, R. E., Polinsky, J., et al. (1987). The genetic defect causing familial Alzheimer's disease maps on chromosome 21. *Science, 235,* 885–890.

Stone, J. H. (1987). Alzheimer's disease and related disorders association. In G. G. Maddox (Ed.), *The encyclopedia of aging* (p. 30). New York: Springer Publishing Co.

Streib, G., & Schneider, C. J. (1971). *Retirement in American society.* Ithaca, NY: Cornell University Press.

Summers, W. K., Majovski, L. V., Marsh, G. M., Tachiki, K., & Kling, A. (1986). Oral tetrahydroaminoacridine in longterm treatment of senile dementia, Alzheimer type. *New England Journal of Medicine, 315,* 1241–1245.

Talbott, J. A., Hales, R. E., & Yudofsky, S.C. (Eds.). (1988). *The American psychiatric press textbook of psychiatry.* Washington, DC: American Psychiatric Press.

Taylor, I. A. (1974). Patterns of creativity and aging. In E. Pfeiffer (Ed.), *Successful aging.* Duke University, Durham, NC: Center for the Study of Aging and Human Development.

Teri, L., Larson, E. B., & Reifler, B. V. (1988). Behavioral disturbance in dementia of the Alzheimer's type. *Journal of the American Geriatrics Society, 36,* 1–6.

Terry, R. D. (1985). Some unanswered questions about the mechanisms and etiology of Alzheimer's disease. *Danish Medical Bulletin, 32* (Supplement 1), 22–24.

Terry, R. D., & Davies, P. (1983). Some morphologic and biochemical aspects of Alzheimer's disease. In D. Samuel, S. Algeri, S. Gershon, V. E. Brimm, & G. Toffano (Eds.), *Aging of the brain.* New York: Raven Press.

Thomae, H. (1980). Personality and adjustment to aging. In J. E. Birren, & R. B. Sloane (Eds.), *Handbook of mental health and aging.* Englewood Cliffs, NJ: Prentice-Hall.

Thomas, L. (1981). On the problem of dementia. *Discover, 2,* 34.

Tice, R. R., & Setlow, R. B. (1985). DNA repair and replication in aging organisms and cells. In C. E. Finch, & E. L. Schneider (Eds.), *Handbook of the biology of aging* (2nd ed.). New York: Van Nostrand Reinhold.

Tonna, E. A. (1977). Aging of skeletal-dental systems and supporting tissues. In C. E. Finch, & L. Hayflick (Eds.), *Handbook of the biology of aging* (1st ed.). New York: Van Nostrand Reinhold.

Torrance, E. P. (1977). Creativity and the older adult. *The Creative Child and Adult Quarterly, Autumn,* 136–144.

Toynbee, A. (1969). *Experiences.* New York: Oxford University Press.

Twain, M. (1963). Seventieth birthday. In C. Neider (Ed.), *The complete essays of Mark Twain.* Garden City, NY: Doubleday & Co.

U. S. Congress, Office of Technology Assessment. (1987). *Losing a million minds Confronting the tragedy of Alzheimer's disease and other dementias.* Washington, DC: U. S. Government Printing Office OTA-BA-323.

U. S. Department of Health and Human Services. (1987). Differential diagnosis of dementing disorders. *National Institutes of Health Consensus Development Statement, 6* (11), 1–27.

U. S. Department of Health and Human Services. (1984). *Report of the Secretary's Task Force on Alzheimer's Disease* (DHHS Publication No. (ADM) 84-1323). Washington, DC: U. S. Government Printing Office.

U. S. Department of Health and Human Services. (1982). *Depression and manic-depressive illness* (NIH publication No. 82-1940). Bethesda, MD: Clinical Center Office of Clinical Reports & Inquiries.

U. S. Senate Committee on Aging. (1984). *Aging America: Trends and projections.* Washington, DC: U. S. Senate Committee on Aging in Conjunction with the American Association of Retired Persons.

Veith, R. C., & Raskind, M. A. (1988). The neurobiology of aging: Does it predispose to depression? *Neurobiology Of Aging, 9,* 101–117.

Verwoerdt, A. (1980). Anxiety, dissociative and personality disorders in the elderly. In E. W. Busse, & Dan G. Blazer (Eds.), *Handbook of Geriatric Psychiatry.* New York: Van Nostrand Reinhold.

Verwoerdt, A. (1981). Individual psychotherapy in senile dementia. In N. E. Miller, & G. D. Cohen (Eds.), *Clinical aspects of Alzheimer's disease and senile dementia.* New York: Raven Press.

Verwoerdt, A., Pfeiffer, E., & Wang, H. (1970). Sexual behavior in senescence. In E. Palmore (Ed.), *Normal aging.* Durham, NC: Duke University Press.

Vestal, R. E. (1985). Clinical pharmacology. In R. Andres, E. Bierman, & W. R. Hazzard (Eds.), *Principles of geriatric medicine.* New York: McGraw-Hill.

Walton, K. W. (1978). Atherosclerosis and aging. In J. C. Brocklehurst (Ed.), *Textbook of geriatric medicine and gerontology* (2nd ed.). New York: Churchill Livingstone.

Wang, E. (1985). A 57,000-mol-wt protein uniquely present in nonproliferating cells and senescent human fibroblasts. *Journal of Cell Biology, 100,* 545–551.

Wang, E., & Lin, S. L. (1986). Disappearance of statin, a protein marker for non-proliferating and senescent cells, following serum-stimulated cell cycle entry. *Experimental Cell Research, 167,* 135–143.

Wang, H. S. (1981). Neuropsychiatric procedures for the assessment of Alzheimer's disease, senile dementia, and related disorders. In N. E. Miller, & G. D. Cohen, *Clinical aspects of Alzheimer's disease and senile dementia (Aging,* Vol. 15). New York: Raven Press.

Warner, H. R., Butler, R. N., Sprott, R. L., & Schneider, E. L. (Eds.). (1987). *Modern biological theories of aging.* New York: Raven Press.

Weinberg, J. (1974). What do I say to my mother when I have nothing to say? *Geriatrics, 29* (11).

Weinberg, J. (1976). On adding insight to injury. *Gerontologist, 16,* 4–10.

Weiner, H. (1985). Schizophrenia: Etiology. In H. I. Kaplan, & B. J. Sadock (Eds.), *Comprehensive textbook of psychiatry/IV* (Vol. 1). Baltimore, MD: Williams & Wilkins.

Weissman, M. M., & Boyd, J. H. (1985). Affective disorders: Epidemiology. In H. I. Kaplan, & B. J. Sadock (Eds.), *Comprehensive textbook of psychiatry/IV* (Vol. 1). Baltimore, MD: Williams & Wilkins.

Wells, C. E. (1982). Refinements in the diagnosis of dementia. *American Journal of Psychiatry, 139,* 621–622.

White, J. A., McGue, M., & Heston, L. L. (1986). Fertility and parental age in Alzheimer's disease. *Journal of Gerontology, 41* (1), 40–43.

White, R. J., Albin, M. S., Locke, G. E., & Davidson, E. (1965). Brain transplantation: Prolonged survival of brain after carotid-jugular interposition. *Science, 150,* 779–781.

Whitehouse, P. J. (1987). Neurotransmitter receptor alterations in Alzheimer's disease: A review. *Alzheimer Disease and Associated Disorders, 1* (1), 9–18.

Whitehouse, P. J., Price, D. L., Clark, A. W., Coyle, J. T., & DeLong, M. R. (1981). Alzheimer disease: Evidence for selective loss of cholinergic neurons in the nucleus basalis. *Annals of Neurology, 10,* 122–126.

Whitlock, F. A., & Siskind, M. (1979). Depression and cancer: A follow-up study. *Psychological Medicine, 9,* 747–752.

Willet, W. C., & MacMahon, B. (1984). Diet and cancer—An overview. *New England Journal of Medicine, 310,* 633–8.

Williams, T. F. (Ed.). (1984). *Rehabilitation in the aging.* New York: Raven Press.

Willis, S. L. (1985). Toward an educational psychology of the older adult learner: Intellectual and cognitive bases. In J. E. Birren, & K. W. Schaie (Eds.), *Handbook of the psychology of aging.* New York: Van Nostrand Reinhold.

Wisniewski, H. M. (1983). Neuritic (senile) and amyloid plaques. In B. Reisberg (Ed.), *Alzheimer's disease: The standard reference.* New York: The Free Press.

Wisniewski, H. M., & Merz, G. S., (1983). Neuritic and amyloid plaques in senile dementia of the Alzheimer type. In R. Katzman (Ed.), *Biological aspects of Alzheimer's disease* (Banbury Report 15). Cold Spring Harbor, NY: Cold Spring Harbor Laboratory.

Wisniewski, K. E., Dalton, A. J., Crapper-McLachlan, D. R., Wen, G. Y., & Wisniewski, H. M. (1985). Alzheimer's disease in Down's syndrome: Clinicopathologic studies. *Neurology, 35,* 957–961.

Wolozin, B. L., Pruchnicki, A., Dickson, D. W., & Davies, P. (1976). A neuronal antigen in the brains of Alzheimer patients. *Science, 232,* 648–650.

Wurtman, R. J. (1985). Alzheimer's disease. *Scientific American, 252,* 62–74.

Yesavage, J. A. (1983). Use of vasoactive medications in the treatment of senile dementia. In B. Reisberg (Ed.), *Alzheimer's disease.* New York: The Free Press.

Yesavage, J. A., & Widrow, L. A. (1985). Senile dementia: psychological and behavioral treatments. In C. M. Gaitz, & T. Samorajski (Eds.), *Aging 2000: our health care destiny, volume I: biomedical issues* (pp. 477–492). New York: Springer-Verlag.

Zarit, S. H., Cole, K. D., & Guider, R. L. (1981). Memory training strategies and subjective complaints of memory in the aged. *The Gerontologist, 21,* 158–164.

Zung, W. W. K. (1980). Affective disorders. In E. W. Busse, & D. G. Blazer (Eds.), *Handbook of geriatric psychiatry.* New York: Van Nostrand Reinhold.

Index